Colonoscopy - Diagnostic and Therapeutic Advances

Edited by Luis Rodrigo

Published in London, United Kingdom

Colonoscopy - Diagnostic and Therapeutic Advances
http://dx.doi.org/10.5772/intechopen.111260
Edited by Luis Rodrigo

Contributors
Luis Rodrigo, Al Aloul Adnan, Varlas Valentin, Kumud S. Altmayer, Arum Linangkung, Umid Kumar Shrestha, Riya Patel, Shivani Patel, Ilyas Momin, Shreeraj Shah

First published in London, United Kingdom, 2024 by IntechOpen
IntechOpen is the global imprint of INTECHOPEN LIMITED, registered in England and Wales, registration number: 11086078, 5 Princes Gate Court, London, SW7 2QJ, United Kingdom

British Library Cataloguing-in-Publication Data
A catalogue record for this book is available from the British Library

Additional hard and PDF copies can be obtained from orders@intechopen.com

Colonoscopy - Diagnostic and Therapeutic Advances
Edited by Luis Rodrigo
p. cm.
Print ISBN 978-0-85466-401-6
Online ISBN 978-0-85466-400-9
eBook (PDF) ISBN 978-0-85466-402-3

For EU product safety concerns:
IN TECH d.o.o., Prolaz Marije Krucifikse Kozulić 3, 51000 Rijeka, Croatia,
info@intechopen.com or visit our website at intechopen.com.

Meet the editor

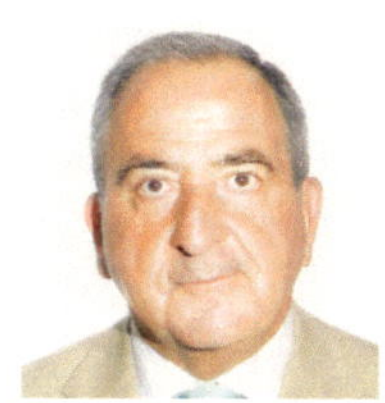

Luis Rodrigo has been a Full Professor of Medicine at the University of Oviedo, Spain, since 2010, and Emeritus Professor since 2014. He is a specialist in gastroenterology and obtained his Ph.D. in 1975. He was appointed Titular Professor in Medicine, University of Oviedo, in 1983. He has been the head of the Gastroenterology Service of the Central University Hospital of Asturias (HUCA), Oviedo, Spain, since 1975. Dr. Rodrigo is the author of eight books on the treatment of gastroenterological and other digestive and liver diseases. He has also authored 58 book chapters and is the author or co-author of 450 scientific papers in English and 282 papers in Spanish.

Contents

Preface

Colonoscopy is the usual endoscopic procedure recommended to examine the large intestine and part of the distal small intestine. It is achieved by introducing a colonoscope, a long, flexible tube-shaped tool with a micro-camera placed at the tip of the endoscope, through the rectum. The colonoscope has several channels inside through which various instruments can be used to facilitate the execution of diagnostic tests and allow the removal of tumors or intestinal polyps.

To perform a colonoscopy, the whole intestine must be completely free of fecal remains. To correctly prepare the colon, a series of laxatives are usually administered, both orally and through enemas, along with the intake of copious amounts of water. Laxatives cause powerful diarrhea that generally cleans the entire colon well and prepares it for the endoscopy.

Colonoscopy is the best test for exploration of the colon, being necessary to examine in detail the walls of both the large and small intestine, the full colon and terminal ileum, and the interior of the lumen. The execution of biopsies and the removal of polyps or tumors is carried out throughout the procedure, both during introduction and withdrawal.

Colonoscopy is indicated for colorectal cancer prophylaxis, diagnosis of the cause of changes in defecation habits, monitoring of patients with ulcerative colitis or Crohn's disease, and diagnosis of unexplained abdominal symptoms.

The usual type of anesthesia used during colonoscopy is sedation. This includes the use of a series of medications that help the patient relax and ensure that the patient does not experience pain or abdominal discomfort. Sedation is usually performed intravenously or by intramuscular injection. Sedation can be superficial or deep. The choice of one type of sedative or another depends on the patient's tolerance to pain and the discomfort inherent to the colonoscopy. It is advisable to administer the lowest degree of sedation possible to be able to perform the exam with the greatest possible reliability while ensuring minimal discomfort for the patient.

A colonoscopy is performed with the patient lying on their side. A specialist is responsible for administering sedation and monitoring vital signs. The exam usually does not begin until the patient is ready and the sedation has taken effect. After thoroughly lubricating the colonoscope, the doctor will insert it through the anus. Progression will be slow and smooth. To facilitate the transit of the colonoscope, carbon dioxide will be blown. The doctor may ask the patient to perform some type of movement as another method to facilitate the movement of the colonoscope. During the examination, the doctor may identify suspicious lesions or polyps. Colonoscopy allows both removal of the polyp and biopsy of the lesion for diagnosis. The colonoscopy itself can last between 20 and 60 minutes. During the test, it may be determined that the colon cleansing before the procedure is not sufficient, and thus, the doctor will stop the colonoscopy and schedule a new appointment.

It takes some time for the effects of sedation to wear off completely. The patient must remain in the clinic for about one to two hours after the colonoscopy. Even so, full recovery usually occurs the next day. This is why it is always recommended that an adult accompany the patient to their colonoscopy. Patients are advised not to drive any type of vehicle or operate heavy machinery on the same day the test is performed.

At the end of the colonoscopy, the doctor may recommend a specific diet for the patient for the next few days. The patient may find blood in their stool after the procedure, but this is common. If the blood in the stool is excessive or lasts too long, the patient will need to contact their doctor.

The process of performing a colonoscopy is safe, but like any other treatment, it may cause some risks or inconveniences. Anal bleeding and colon perforation are the most likely problems, although these complications are rare. Bleeding can occur during the colonoscopy or even two weeks after it is performed. If any of these problems occur, the specialist is in charge of stopping the bleeding. Among the less common drawbacks of colonoscopy are the presence of diverticulitis, anal pain, infections, or abdominal discomfort. Cardiovascular complications may also arise, such as low blood pressure or irregular transitory heartbeats.

This book discusses all these aspects of colonoscopy and more, including the latest innovations and advances achieved in recent years, with a focus on those achieved with the emergence of artificial intelligence (AI).

I want to thank all the chapter authors for their excellent contributions. Special thanks go to Ms. Elvira Baumgartner at IntechOpen for her continuous help and support throughout the editorial process.

Luis Rodrigo MD
University of Oviedo,
Oveido, Spain

Chapter 1

Introductory Chapter: The Actual State of Colonoscopy

Luis Rodrigo

1. Introduction

Before dealing with the characteristics and indications of colonoscopy, let us briefly refer to its younger sister, flexible sigmoidoscopy, which, as its name indicates, is used only for the distal exploration of the colon, including the rectum and sigmoid, which is also interesting to know in its applications that are complementary in some cases, with the complete exploration of the entire colon.

2. Flexible sigmoidoscopy: indications and contraindications

It has been at least two decades since flexible sigmoidoscopy has replaced conventional rectoscopy, and the reasons must be sought independently of the limited associated discomfort and in a better general acceptance of the use of a flexible instrument instead of the introduction of a rigid tube, as well as obtaining greater diagnostic performance in the detection of polyps and/or rectal tumors.

However, with the introduction and progressive development of colonoscopy worldwide, which allows the entire colon and terminal ileum to be adequately explored, sigmoidoscopy has been losing prominence in most clinical centers. However, it still has some indications, which are summarized: 1. Study of the distal pathology of the colon (ano-rectal). 2. Evaluation of cases of acute diarrhea. 3. Monitoring and control of ulcerative colitis. 4. Periodic control of ileo-anal reservoirs. 5. In patients with low tumor risk in asymptomatic patients. 6. In those over 50 years of age, without a family history. 7. In relatives of patients with familial adenomatous polyposis from the age of 10 and annually. 8. In surveillance of the excluded rectal stump in cases of inflammatory bowel disease.

Two absolute contraindications are included: 1. Severe acute diverticulitis. 2. Suspected intestinal perforation.

In United States and some other countries, sigmoidoscopy is usually performed by specialized nurses under the direct supervision and occasional help of expert endoscopists [1].

3. Colonoscopy: indications and contraindications

The development of colonoscopy in recent decades worldwide has followed a course parallel to advances in knowledge of the sequence of changes from polyp to carcinoma in the colon. Malignant colon and rectal tumors are often associated with

IntechOpen

certain conditions that are considered premalignant. In colorectal carcinoma, the most common premalignant lesion consists of the presence of adenomatous polyps. Therefore, the development of an early diagnosis plan is based on the periodic and careful surveillance of patients with premalignant lesions in order to detect the presence of cancers at an early (pre-symptomatic) stage, when endoscopic or surgical cure is still possible. It is possible...

Although there is any conclusive evidence in controlled studies to support that endoscopic surveillance reduces the mortality rate, some data suggest improved survival of patients included in surveillance programs.

Consequently, colonoscopy has acquired maximum notoriety, as has the close control of the evolution of adenomatous polyps. The advance in colonoscopy knowledge regarding the possibility of detecting the presence of premalignant lesions and at the same time, being able to remove them, replacing the opaque enema due to its greater capacity for the diagnosis and treatment of these lesions.

The indications for colonoscopy can be divided into two categories: diagnostic and therapeutic (**Tables 1** and **2**). The contraindications and complications of this technique are also described (**Tables 3–5**) [2–5].

• For the evaluation of repletion defects and/or stenosis, visualized in the Opaque Enema
• First of all, Iron Deficiency Anemia of unexplained origin
• In the evaluation of Gastrointestinal Bleeding of unclear origin
• Melenas with previous normal Esophago-Gastro-Duodenoscopy study
• Confirmed presence of Occult Blood in Feces
• Hematochezia that does not clearly come from the rectum or perianal region
• To rule out synchronous lesions (Cancer and/or Polyps) in patients with these suspicious findings
• Post-resection follow-up of CRC or neoplastic polyps at periodic intervals
• In family screening for hereditary CRC and subsequent follow-up

Table 1.
Indications for diagnostic colonoscopy.

• Treatment of all types of bleeding lesions of the colon (post-polypectomy, angiomas, neoplasms, diverticula, vascular anomalies)
• Removal of foreign bodies from the colon and rectum
• Decompression of acute non-toxic megacolon, or sigmoid volvulus
• Balloon dilation of stenotic lesions
• Removal of colon polyps
• Palliative treatment of tumorous, stenotic, or bleeding lesions
• Bridging treatment prior to surgery of colonic obstructions secondary to malignant lesions

Table 2.
Indications for therapeutic colonoscopy.

• Chronic Abdominal Pain and Irritable Bowel Syndrome that does not present diagnostic doubts
• Acute self-limited diarrhea
• Routine monitoring of inflammatory bowel disease
• Digestive bleeding of known cause in the upper digestive tract
• Acute fulminant colitis
• Acute diverticulitis
• Acute pancreatitis
• Recent postoperative colonic surgery
• Second and third trimester of pregnancy
• When the risks to the patient's health and/or life are greater than the benefits of the examination
• Suspected perforation of a hollow viscus
• In patients with recent pulmonary embolism
• When there is no collaboration on the part of the patient

Table 3.
Contraindications of colonoscopy.

• Bacteremia
• Drilling
• Pneumatic drilling
• Hemorrhage
• Volvulus
• Cardiac and/or ECG alterations
• Aortic aneurysm dissection
• Post-colonoscopy distention syndrome
• Vaso-vagal reflex
• Incarceration of an inguinal hernia
• Impaction of the endoscope into the hernial sac

Table 4.
Complications of diagnostic colonoscopy.

• Hemorrhage
• Drilling
• Incomplete polypectomy
• Post-polypectomy syndrome (suffering of the colon wall due to excess coagulation)
• Exitus

Table 5.
Complications of therapeutic colonoscopy.

4. Preparation and cleaning of the colon for performing the colonoscopy

It is carried out through the ingestion of an electrolyte solution of polyethylene glycol (PEG) with electrolyte solution at a rate of 250 cc orally every 15 minutes, up to a total of 2-3 liters. It can be used safely in patients with heart, kidney, and liver diseases, as it prevents dehydration and significant loss of electrolytes, its main disadvantage being the large amount of liquid that the patient has to drink and its salty taste, which can induce vomiting, in up to 10% of cases. It is possible to administer a prokinetic such as cisapride at a dose of 20 mg. Thirty minutes before starting to take the preparation, reduce the chances of nausea and/or vomiting.

The Fleet preparation is also recommended, which obtains similar results to the PEG/electrolyte solution preparation, probably with greater acceptance by patients, since the volume of the solution to be ingested is smaller, only 90 ml., followed by abundant amount of liquid to choose for each patient. Its main drawback is the risk of dehydration and the appearance of hydroelectrolyte alterations, being contraindicated in patients with associated diseases. Another possible side effect of this preparation is the appearance of thrush-type mucosal lesions in the colon, which can be misleading and appear in up to 15% of cases [6–8].

5. Preparation in special situations

5.1 Persistent constipation

If there is evidence of chronic constipation, it is suggested to always indicate intense bowel preparation. It is advisable to administer an effective oral purgative the day before, along with the intake of large quantities of liquids.

5.2 Colostomy wearers

It is as difficult to prepare as normal colon, so the usual preparation should not be modified.

5.3 Ileal reservoirs

These patients should be prepared with saline enemas and repeated until they come out completely clean.

5.4 Conventional ileostomy

They do not require preparation.

5.5 Ileorectal anastomosis

Administration of a saline enema is usually sufficient.

5.6 "Shotgun barrel" colostomy

The distal loop of a shotgun colostomy usually contains a considerable amount of viscous mucus and some thick debris that can block the colonoscope. For all these reasons, it is recommended to introduce a water/saline enema or lavage through the colostomy, before examining an intestine devoid of function.

5.7 Inflammatory bowel disease

Patients with severe colitis rarely need a colonoscopy, since a simple abdominal X-ray usually provides sufficient information, making its performance largely contraindicated.

In cases of moderate or mild colitis, the preparation should be the usual one with PEG solutions, balanced with electrolytes.

5.8 Treatment with oral iron preparations

Its administration must be suspended at least 7 days before performing the examination.

5.9 Antiplatelet or anticoagulated patients

There is no evidence that continued low-dose aspirin may increase the risk of bleeding after polypectomy, and therefore, this medication does not need to be discontinued.

In anticoagulated with warfarin due to risk of embolism, the medication can be safely suspended 3-4 days before the test, while if the risk is high, due to the presence of metallic heart valves, prior admission of the patient and conversion to heparin, at least 3 hours before the examination.

5.10 Technical aspects related to colonoscopy

The insertion of the colonoscope is a technique that is difficult to teach because, in essence, it consists of introducing a flexible tube, which is the endoscope, through a long and flexible duct, which is the colon.

The latter is characterized by having a variable length, mobility, and fixation, its movements being unpredictable after the introduction of the endoscope inside.

Since the colon is an elastic tube, it becomes arduous and tortuous with air insufflation, with the frequent formation of loops and angulations after its dilation. However, when deflated, it is much shorter. The following principles must be observed when performing a colonoscopy:

1. Insufflate the minimum amount of air throughout the entire examination and aspirate it whenever possible.

2. Avoid the formation of loops (for which you have to push as little as possible).

3. Move the endoscope back, with the aim of shortening the colon whenever possible, inserting it according to the anatomical position in which the viewer is located, 40 cm in the descending colon and inserted, in the splenic angle of 50 cm, transverse colon of about 60 cm, being at the level of the cecum, 70-80 cm.

4. Monitor at all times the presence of discomfort that the patient presents, which indicates excessive insufflation, or the formation of loops, trying to rectify the position of the endoscope if this occurs.

5. If the tip of the endoscope does not advance, try different combinations of changes, including patient posture, instrument pressure, and tube rotation.

Unassisted colonoscopy is recommended as the ideal method and is performed by most experienced endoscopists. This method requires discipline of the hands, and it is recommended that each hand have a certain task. Thus, while the left hand is in charge of holding the colonoscope and manages the air, water and aspiration controls and the up-down control and only on some occasions in the lateral control. The right hand is used to twist the instrument and becomes an essential part of the exploration [9, 10].

There are three different kinds of rotational effects:

a. Rotation with the endoscope and the straight tip is done by rotating the instrument on its axis. This movement can be used to orient the biopsy forceps, adhere the polypectomy loop to a specific lesion, or to position the aspiration channel precisely over a fluid accumulator.

b. Rotation with the endoscope straight and the tip angled and directed upwards, clockwise twisting deviates it to the right, while with the tip directed downwards, the same clockwise movement produces a deviation to the left.

c. Rotation with a loop is usually formed at the sigmoid level. To try to resolve it, it is advisable to perform a clockwise rotation, so that the mobile sigmoid is shortened above the endoscope, while the end of the latter will ascend toward the fixed ascending colon.

6. Colonoscopy with magnification and chromography

In recent years, a very important development has been achieved in video image quality, since chips (> 400,000 pixels) have been incorporated into colonoscopes that produce high-resolution images that are digitally treated, thus achieving greater definition (similar to that obtained using low-power microscopes with 100× image magnification) [11].

This technique, together with the staining of the mucosa using dyes, allows us to better visualize its surface and thus differentiate between those neoplastic polyps and those that are not.

Furthermore, Chromography and Endoscopic Magnification are also useful when applied to follow-up [12].

For patients with long-standing ulcerative colitis, since staining the mucosa with dyes such as methylene blue allows us to detect areas of possible dysplasia and direct biopsy taking toward them.

Author details

Luis Rodrigo
University of Oviedo, Spain

*Address all correspondence to: lrodrigosaez@gmail.com

References

[1] Chengren Z, Lili L, Li J, et al. Effect of flexible sigmoidoscopy-based screening on colorectal cancer incidence and mortality: An updated systematic review and meta-analysis of randomized controlled trials. Expert Review of Anticancer Therapy. 2023;**23**:1217-1227

[2] Hassan C, Piovani D, Spadaccini M, et al. Variability in adenoma detection rate in control groups of randomized colonoscopy trials: A systematic review and meta-analysis. Gastrointestinal Endoscopy. 2023;**97**:212-225

[3] Ishibashi F, Suzuki S, Nagai M, et al. Colorectal cold snare polypectomy: Current standard technique and future perspective. Digestive Endoscopy. 2023;**35**:278-286

[4] Spadaccini M, Scilliro A, Sharma P, Repici A, Hassan C, Voza A. Adenoma detection rate in colonoscopy: How can it be improved? Expert Review of Gastroenterology & Hepatology. 2023;**17**(11):1089-1099

[5] Spada C, Hassan C, Bellini D, et al. Imaging alternatives to colonoscopy: CT colonography and colon capsule. European society of gastrointestinal endoscopy (ESGE) and European society of gastrointestinal and abdominal radiology (ESGAR) guideline update 2020. Endoscopy. 2020;**52**:1127-1141

[6] Gimeno-García AZ, Benítez-Zafra F, Nicolás-Pérez D, Hernández-Guerra M. Colon bowel preparation in the era of artificial intelligence: Is there potential for enhancing colon bowel cleansing? Medicina (Kaunas, Lithuania). 2023;**59**:1834

[7] Rosa B, Donato H, Cúrdia Gonçalves T, Sousa-Pinto B, Cotter J. What is the optimal bowel preparation for capsule colonoscopy and pan-intestinal capsule endoscopy? A systematic review and meta-analysis. Digestive Diseases and Sciences. 2023;**68**:4418-431. DOI: 10.1007/s10620-023-08133-7

[8] Kametaka D, Ito M, Kawano S, et al. Optimal bowel preparation method to visualize the distal ileum via small bowel capsule endoscopy. Diagnostics (Basel). 2023;**13**:3269

[9] Gornick D, Kadakuntla A, Trovato A, Stetzer R, Tadros M. Practical considerations for colorectal cancer screening in older adults. World Journal of Gastrointestinal Oncology. 2022;**14**:1086-1102

[10] Herman T, Megna B, Pallav K, Bilal M. Endoscopic mucosal resection: Tips and tricks for gastrointestinal trainees. Translational Gastroenterology and Hepatology. 2023;**8**:25

[11] Teramoto A, Hamada S, Ogino B, Yasuda I, Sano Y. Updates in narrow-band imaging for colorectal polyps: Narrow-band imaging generations, detection, diagnosis, and artificial intelligence. Digestive Endoscopy. 2023;**35**:453-470

[12] Almeida R, Lopez F, Rocha P, et al. Polyp detection in the cecum and ascending colon by dye based chromoendoscopy is its routine use justified? Revista do Colégio Brasileiro de Cirurgiões. 2023;**50**:e20233562

Chapter 2

Colorectal Cancer: Colonoscopy and Follow Up

Al Aloul Adnan and Varlas Valentin

Abstract

Pelvic recurrence is a significant concern following curative resection for rectal cancer, regardless of the tumor's origin of the rectum. In this retrospective observational study, 219 patients were analyzed, with 213 undergoing surgical treatment for rectal cancer at three surgical centers between 2014 and 2019. Surgical procedures included anterior resection with Hartmann's procedure (39 patients), anterior resection of rectosigmoid with colorectal anastomosis (130 cases), and abdominoperineal resection (44 cases). After a 2-year follow-up, pelvic recurrence occurred in 19 patients, constituting approximately 8.9% of cases. The recurrence rates varied among surgical procedures, with a 15.38% recurrence rate after the Hartmann procedure, 9% after abdominoperineal resection, and 7% after anterior resection of rectosigmoid with colorectal anastomosis. Emphasize the high recurrence rates associated with advanced stages of rectal cancer. Notably, its follow-up was done clinically, by laboratory tests, colonoscopy (the main test for pelvic recurrence) after 6 months of surgery, 12 months, and 2 years, computed tomography (CT), magnetic resonance imaging (MRI), and pelvic ultrasound at one year and 2 years, a lower recurrence rate being indicative of a successful curative surgical treatment. The Hartmann procedure, often performed as an emergency operation for locally advanced lesions, exhibited the highest recurrence rate.

Keywords: pelvic recurrence, rectal cancer, colonoscopy, future direction, anastomasis

1. Introduction

A colonoscopy is a medical procedure used to examine the inside of the colon and rectum. It is an essential tool for diagnosing and monitoring various gastrointestinal conditions, including colorectal cancer, inflammatory bowel disease, and polyps.

Space of endoscopy rooms: reception and waiting room, room procedure, (**Figure 1**), recovery room, postprocedural and consultation room, and the last training room for students and residents. Equipment: endoscope tower – endoscope, monitor, insufflation, light source, and other instruments that are necessary for procedures, storage instruments, accessories, and consumables. The control of infection is carried out by cleaning and sterilization room.

Here's a brief overview of the colonoscopy procedure:

1.1 Preparation

Before the colonoscopy, patients are instructed to follow a specific diet and bowel preparation regimen. This often involves following a clear liquid diet and taking a laxative or bowel-cleansing solution to empty the colon.

1.2 Arrival at the medical facility

Patients typically arrive at a hospital or an outpatient clinic for the procedure. They will be asked to change into a hospital gown.

Consent form and Medical History. You will be asked to sign a consent form, and a nurse or healthcare provider will review medical history, including any allergies, medications you're currently taking, and any pre-existing medical conditions.

Sedation and monitoring: Most colonoscopies are performed with sedation or anesthesia to ensure the patient's comfort and minimize discomfort. The patient is closely monitored throughout the procedure, including vital signs like blood pressure, heart rate, and oxygen levels.

Positioning: The patient will be positioned on your left side on an examination table. *of the colonoscope:* A long, flexible tube colonoscope is inserted through the anus and advanced slowly into the colon until cecum and ileocecal valve. The colonoscope has a light and a camera at the tip, allowing the doctor to view the inner lining of the colon on a monitor.

Examination of the colon: As the colonoscope is advanced, the examiner views the entire length of the colon, looking for abnormalities, such as polyps, inflammation, diverticula, or tumors. *Biopsy or polyps removal (if necessary):* During the colonoscopy, the endoscopist may take tissue samples (biopsies) if suspicious areas are found. Additionally, small polyps can often be removed during the procedure to prevent them from becoming cancerous [1].

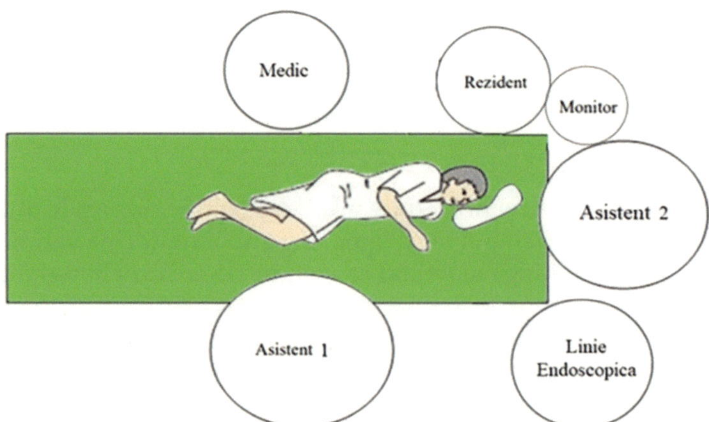

Figure 1.
Colonoscopy position.

Documentation: After a thorough examination, the colonoscope is slowly withdrawn, and the endoscopist carefully documents any findings. This documentation may include photographs or video recordings.

Recovery: After the colonoscopy, patients are taken to a recovery area where they can rest and recover from the sedation. It's essential to have a friend or family member available to drive the patient home because the sedation can temporarily impair judgment and coordination. *Post-procedure discussion:* Once the patient is fully awake and alert, the endoscopist and nurse will discuss the findings of the colonoscopy with the patient. If biopsies were taken, results may not be available immediately and could take a few days.

Follow-up and recommendations: Depending on the results of the colonoscopy, the doctor may recommend further tests or treatments. Patients may also receive guidance on lifestyle changes, such as dietary adjustments or regular screenings.

2. Types of screening tests

Stool tests: Guaiac-based fecal occult blood test (gFOBT): This test uses the chemical guaiac to detect blood in stool. At home, you could use a stick or brush to obtain a small amount of stool. You then return the test sample to the healthcare provider or a laboratory, where stool samples are checked for blood. Fecal immunochemical test (FIT): This test uses antibodies to detect blood in the stool. You receive a test kit from your healthcare provider. This test is done the same way as gFOBT. FIT-DNA test: (or stool DNA test) This test combines the FIT with a test to detect altered DNA in stool [2]. You collect a test sample to check for an entire bowel movement and send it to a laboratory to be tested for cancer cells.

Flexible sigmoidoscopy (Flex Sig): The healthcare provider puts a short, thin, flexible, lighted tube into your rectum and checks for polyps or cancer inside the rectum and lower third of the colon.

Colonoscopy: Similar to flexible sigmoidoscopy, except the healthcare provider uses a longer, thin, flexible, lighted tube to check for polyps or cancer inside the rectum and the entire colon. During the test, the healthcare provider can find and remove most polyps and some cancers. Colonoscopy may also be used as a follow-up test if one of the other screening tests finds anything unusual.

CT colonography (virtual colonoscopy): Computed tomography (CT) colonography, also called a virtual colonoscopy, uses X-rays and computers to produce images of the entire colon. The images are displayed on a computer screen for the healthcare provider to analyze.

DNA stool tests, such as Cologuard, detect specific DNA changes associated with colorectal cancer.

Colorectal cancer follow-up colonoscopy: Follow-up colonoscopies are an essential part of monitoring individuals who have previously been diagnosed with colorectal cancer or who have had precancerous polyps removed during a colonoscopy. The specific recommendations for follow-up colonoscopies can vary based on the individual's medical history, the stage of cancer, and the presence of any risk factors [3].

However, here is a general guideline for follow-up colonoscopies after a colorectal cancer diagnosis:

Posttreatment evaluation: After the initial diagnosis and treatment of colorectal cancer, your healthcare provider will typically recommend a follow-up evaluation to assess the effectiveness of the treatment and to check for any signs of cancer recurrence.

3. Importance of early detection

Improved survival rates: When colorectal cancer is detected at an early stage, the chances of successful treatment and long-term survival are significantly higher. In fact, for localized colorectal cancer (cancer that hasn't spread beyond the colon or rectum), the 5-year survival rate can exceed 90%. Early detection allows for timely intervention and more effective treatment options. Minimized treatment intensity: Early stage colorectal cancer often requires less aggressive treatment than advanced-stage cancer. Surgery alone may be curative in many cases, sparing patients from the need for extensive chemotherapy or radiation therapy. Early detection can prevent the cancer from progressing to a more advanced stage, which may involve more invasive treatments and potentially debilitating symptoms, and this helps in maintaining a better quality of life for patients [4]. Treating colorectal cancer at an early stage is generally less costly than treating advanced-stage cancer. This can lead to cost savings for patients and healthcare systems.

Prevention of metastasis: Colorectal cancer that is caught early is less likely to metastasize to other organs or lymph nodes. Early detection often allows for the preservation of more of the colon or rectum during surgery, minimizing the need for extensive surgical procedures, such as colostomy or ileostomy [5]. Colorectal cancer often starts as benign growths—polyps. During a colonoscopy, these polyps can be identified and removed, effectively preventing cancer from developing.

The identification of hereditary conditions, such as Lynch syndrome or familial adenomatous polyposis (FAP), which increase the risk of colorectal cancer is important. Identifying these conditions in one family member can lead to early screening and preventive measures for other family members. Screening can detect cancer in its earliest stages or identify precancerous lesions, reducing the overall burden of the disease. Early detection allows for long-term surveillance and monitoring of individuals at higher risk for colorectal cancer. This ensures that any new polyps or cancerous growths are detected promptly.

Initial follow-up colonoscopy: The first follow-up colonoscopy is usually scheduled within the first year after the completion of your initial treatment. The timing may vary depending on the stage and aggressiveness of the cancer (**Figures 2** and **3**).

Frequency of follow-up colonoscopies: The frequency of follow-up colonoscopies after the initial posttreatment evaluation will depend on several factors, including the stage of cancer, the completeness of initial treatment, and individual risk factors. Common recommendations are as follows: High-risk situations (e.g., advanced cancer, positive lymph nodes, or incomplete resection): Colonoscopy every 3–6 months for the first 2–3 years. Intermediate-risk situations: Colonoscopy every 6–12 months for the first 2–3 years. Low-risk situations: Colonoscopy every 1–3 years after the initial follow-up.

Long-term surveillance:

After several years of regular follow-up colonoscopies with no signs of cancer recurrence, the interval between colonoscopies may be extended, typically to every 3–5 years. However, the specific schedule should be determined by your healthcare provider based on your individual case.

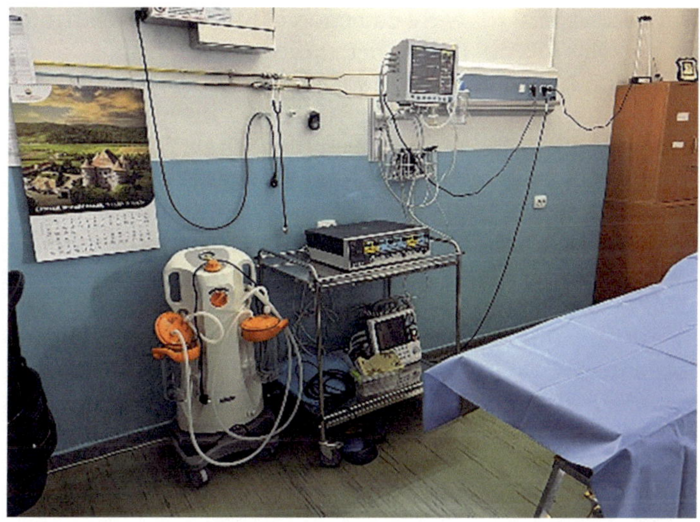

Figure 2.
Recovery room.

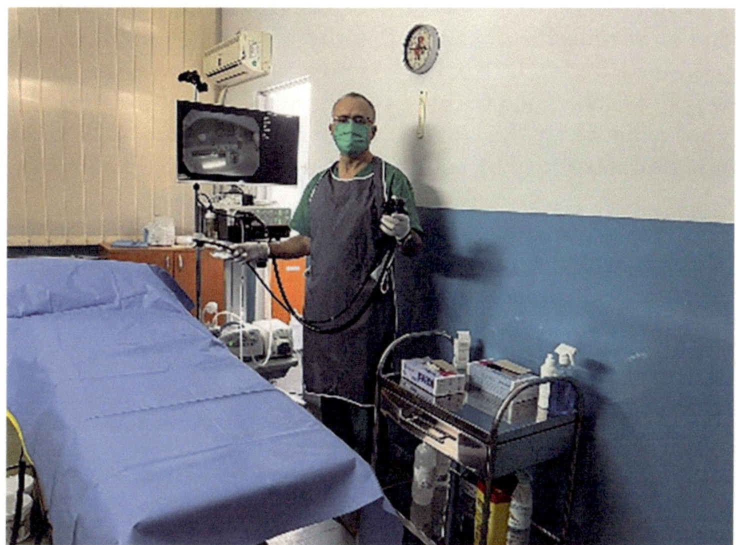

Figure 3.
Room procedure.

4. Lifelong surveillance

In some cases, individuals with a history of colorectal cancer may require lifelong surveillance to monitor for cancer recurrence or the development of new polyps.

Additional testing: In addition to colonoscopy, other tests may be recommended as part of your follow-up, such as blood tests to monitor tumor markers, CT scans, or other imaging studies to check for metastasis (spread of cancer), and regular physical examinations [6].

Adherence to recommendations: It's crucial to adhere to your healthcare provider's recommended follow-up schedule and undergo any additional testing as advised.

Regular follow-up is essential for early detection of any cancer recurrence or new polyps, as early intervention can lead to better outcomes.

Lifestyle and health maintenance: In addition to medical follow-up, maintaining a healthy lifestyle, including a balanced diet, regular exercise, and avoidance of tobacco and excessive alcohol consumption, can help reduce the risk of cancer recurrence and other health problems. Follow-up for rectal cancer typically involves a combination of medical evaluations, imaging studies, and endoscopic procedures to monitor for cancer recurrence and assess the effectiveness of treatment. The specific follow-up plan may vary depending on the stage of cancer, the type of treatment received, and individual patient factors [7].

Here's a general guideline for follow-up after rectal cancer treatment, including endoscopic procedures:

Initial posttreatment evaluation: After completing treatment for rectal cancer, you will undergo an initial evaluation to assess the response to treatment and ensure there is no immediate evidence of cancer recurrence.

This evaluation may include physical examinations, blood tests, and imaging studies such as CT scans.

Endoscopic follow-up procedures: Endoscopic procedures like sigmoidoscopy or colonoscopy are essential for monitoring the rectal area and the rest of the colon for any signs of cancer recurrence or new polyps. The frequency and timing of these procedures depend on various factors, including the stage of the initial cancer, the type of treatment received, and individual risk factors [8]. In some cases, the first follow-up endoscopy may be scheduled within a few months after completing treatment. Subsequent endoscopies may then be performed at regular intervals. The specific schedule should be determined by your healthcare provider based on your individual case (**Figure 4**).

In addition to endoscopy, imaging studies such as CT scans may be recommended periodically to check for any signs of cancer recurrence or metastasis to nearby lymph

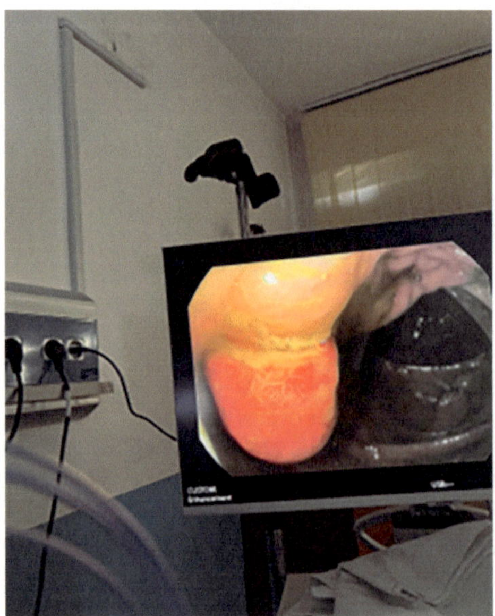

Figure 4.
Local recurrence at enterocolic anastomosis end-side.

nodes or distant organs. Tumor marker testing: Blood tests to monitor tumor markers (e.g., CEA—carcinoembryonic antigen) may be part of your follow-up plan. Elevated levels of these markers can sometimes indicate cancer recurrence. Stool testing: Periodic stool testing for blood or other markers may be recommended to check for any signs of rectal cancer recurrence or new growths. Long-term surveillance: The frequency of follow-up examinations and tests may decrease over time if there are no signs of cancer recurrence. After several years of surveillance with no issues, follow-up intervals may be extended [9]. Adherence to recommendations: It's crucial to adhere to your healthcare provider's recommended follow-up schedule and undergo any necessary tests and procedures. Regular follow-up is essential for early detection of any cancer recurrence or new growths. Lifestyle and health maintenance: Maintaining a healthy lifestyle, including a balanced diet, regular exercise, and avoiding tobacco and excessive alcohol consumption, can help reduce the risk of cancer recurrence and improve overall health.

5. Colonoscopy in colorectal cancer diagnosis

The colonoscope is inserted via anus to rectum and advanced through all of the colon until the cecum, and terminal ileum. The colonoscope inspects the entire mucosa of any lesions—tumors, polyps, ulcerations, or diverticula. Suspicion of any lesion observed may take the specimen for histopathology analyses, which is an important step to confirm the diagnosis. Assess the size, type, and location of the lesions from the anal orifice and this is an important information for the treatment.

The diagnosis of neoplasm after colorectal treatment as local recurrence and new polyps or tumors is used by colonoscopy follow-up for surveillance and monitoring. The screening for tumors and other lesions like inflammatory bowel disease, diverticulosis and diverticulitis, and bleeding is carried out [10].

Staging of colorectal cancer by endoscopy, CT scan, and MRI: The staging of colorectal cancer follows TNM conform to American Joint committee on Cancer (AJCC): (T) tumor size and extent of the primary tumor, (N) lymph nodes that contain malignant cells, and (M) metastasis to distant organs or tissues. The overview of stages of colorectal cancer is given as follows:

Stage 0: (Tis, N0, M0): carcinoma *in situ*. Cancer is confined to the innermost layer of the colon or rectum and has not invaded deeper layers. It has not spread to lymph nodes or distant sites.

Stage I (T1-T2, N0, M0): Cancer has grown through the mucosa and into the submucosa (T1) or muscularis propria (T2) of the colon or rectum. It has not spread to lymph nodes or distant sites.

Stage II Stage IIA (T3, N0, M0): Cancer has penetrated the submucosa and has grown into the muscularis propria (T3) of the colon or rectum. It has not spread to lymph nodes or distant sites. Stage IIB (T4a, N0, M0): Cancer has invaded through the serosa (the outermost layer) of the colon or rectum (T4a). It has not spread to lymph nodes or distant sites. Stage IIC (T4b, N0, M0): Cancer has invaded nearby structures or organs (T4b). It has not spread to lymph nodes or distant sites.

Stage III (Any T, N1/N2, M0): Cancer has invaded lymph nodes (N1/N2) but has not spread to distant sites. This stage is further subdivided into IIIA, IIIB, and IIIC based on the extent of lymph node involvement.

Stage IV (Any T, Any N, M1): Cancer has spread to distant organs or tissues, such as the liver, lungs, and peritoneum. This stage is considered advanced or metastatic colorectal cancer [11].

6. Treatment options for colorectal cancer

Surgery:

Surgical treatment is the most important treatment for colorectal cancer for stage 0 to stage III by endoscopic, laparoscopic, or open approach.

Polypectomy: Removal of small, benign polyps and tumors involved just mucosa during a colonoscopy. Local excision: Removal of small, early stage cancers without affecting a significant portion of the colon or rectum.

Segmental colectomy: Removal of the portion of the colon with lymphadenectomy in V shape the tip of V is to mesentery. The remaining healthy sections are anastomosed.

Right or left hemicolectomy with lymphadenectomy and anastomosis with or without protection.

Anterior resection with primary anastomosis, anterior resection with Hartmann procedure, with end left-sided colostomy.

Abdominoperineal resection with end colostomy for rectal cancer low situation below 4 cm from the anal orifice.

Total colectomy: Removal of the entire colon with enterorectal or anal anastomosis with ileostomy protection of synchronous multiple tumors in the rectum and colon [12].

Surgery may also be used to remove metastatic lesions in other organs, such as the liver (atypical lobectomy) or lungs.

Chemotherapy:

Chemotherapy involves the use of drugs to destroy malignant cells or inhibit their growth and division. Neoadjuvant treatment can be used before surgery, adjuvant after surgery, or as the primary treatment for advanced colorectal cancer (Stage III or IV).

Combination chemotherapy regimens are often used, including drugs like 5-fluorouracil (5-FU), capecitabine, oxaliplatin, and irinotecan [13].

Targeted therapies, such as cetuximab and bevacizumab, may be added to chemotherapy for specific cases.

Radiation therapy:

Radiation therapy uses high-energy X-rays and it may be used in combination with chemotherapy (chemoradiation) to shrink tumors before surgery to treat rectal cancer.

Radiation therapy can also relieve symptoms in advanced cases by shrinking tumors that are causing obstruction or bleeding.

Targeted therapy: Targeted therapies are drugs that specifically target certain molecules or pathways involved in cancer growth. These therapies may be used in combination with chemotherapy for advanced colorectal cancer. Examples include cetuximab, panitumumab, and regorafenib.

Immunotherapy: Immunotherapy, given with drugs such as pembrolizumab or nivolumab, is used in some advanced colorectal cancers with specific biomarkers (e.g., microsatellite instability-high or mismatch repair deficiency). Immunotherapy helps the immune system recognize and attack malignant cells [14].

Palliative care: Palliative care focuses on providing relief from symptoms and improving the quality of life for patients with advanced or metastatic colorectal cancer. It includes pain management, symptom control, and emotional support [15].

6.1 Follow-up colonoscopy

The first follow-up colonoscopy is usually scheduled within the first year after the completion of your initial treatment. The timing may vary depending on the stage and aggressiveness of the cancer.

Common recommendations are as follows: High-risk situations (e.g., advanced cancer, positive lymph nodes, or incomplete resection): Colonoscopy every 3–6 months for the first 2–3 years. Intermediate risk: Colonoscopy every 6–12 months for the first 2–3 years. Low risk: Colonoscopy every 1–3 years after the initial follow-up.

7. Advances in colonoscopy technology

High-definition (HD) and high-resolution imaging: Modern colonoscopes are equipped with high-definition and high-resolution imaging systems. These systems provide clearer and more detailed images of the colon's lining, making it easier to detect abnormalities, such as polyps or early stage cancers.

Narrow-band imaging (NBI): NBI is an optical enhancement technology that uses narrow-bandwidth light to enhance the visualization of blood vessels and mucosal patterns in the colon. This can help differentiate between benign and potentially malignant lesions.

Chromoendoscopy: Chromoendoscopy involves spraying a special dye or contrast agent onto the colon's lining to highlight abnormalities. This technique can improve the detection of small or flat polyps and early stage cancers.

Cap-assisted colonoscopy: A soft, flexible cap can be attached to the tip of the colonoscope to help improve the view of the colon's inner lining. This can be especially helpful in navigating through difficult or tortuous sections of the colon.

Third-eye retroscope: This additional, miniaturized camera at the tip of the colonoscope provides a backward view, enhancing the ability to detect lesions hidden behind folds in the colon.

Wide-angle colonoscopes: Some colonoscopes have a wider field of view, which can help healthcare providers see more of the colon's surface in a single view, reducing the need for excessive maneuvering.

Disposable colonoscopes: Disposable colonoscopes are emerging as an option for reducing the risk of cross-contamination of infection in healthcare settings.

Improved bowel preparation: Innovations in bowel preparation solutions and techniques are making the cleansing process more patient-friendly and effective, ensuring a clearer view during the procedure.

Patient comfort enhancements: Advances in colonoscopy equipment and techniques aim to improve patient comfort. Smaller-diameter scopes, more flexible instruments, and improved sedation options can lead to a more comfortable experience.

Wireless capsule colonoscopy: While not a replacement for traditional colonoscopy, wireless capsule endoscopy allows for the visualization of the colon using a small, ingestible camera capsule. This technology is still evolving and primarily used in specific clinical situations [16].

8. Future directions and research

Personalized medicine and precision oncology: Research is exploring ways to tailor colorectal cancer treatment to the individual patient's specific genetic and molecular profile. Identifying specific mutations and biomarkers in tumors can help determine the most effective targeted therapies and immunotherapies.

Immunotherapy advances: Immunotherapy advances have shown promise in treating some colorectal cancers, particularly those with specific genetic features like microsatellite instability-high or mismatch repair deficiency. Future research aims to expand the use of immunotherapy and identify additional patient subgroups that may benefit.

Early detection and screening: Ongoing research is focused on developing more accurate and less invasive methods for early detection of colorectal cancer and precancerous lesions. This includes blood-based biomarkers, liquid biopsies, and advanced imaging techniques [17, 18].

Artificial intelligence (AI) and machine learning: AI and machine learning algorithms are being developed to assist in the early detection and characterization of colorectal cancer lesions from medical imaging, such as colonoscopy and CT scans.

Minimally invasive surgery: Advances in surgical techniques, including robotics and laparoscopy, are aimed at reducing the invasiveness of colorectal cancer surgery, shortening recovery times, and improving outcomes.

Biomarker discovery: Research continues to identify new biomarkers in blood, tissue, and stool samples that can aid in early diagnosis, prognosis, and treatment selection.

Genetic counseling and testing: Research into genetic risk factors and hereditary syndromes is ongoing. Identifying at-risk individuals and providing appropriate genetic counseling and testing can help with early intervention and risk reduction.

Targeted therapies: Investigational targeted therapies are being developed to target specific signaling pathways involved in colorectal cancer growth. Research is ongoing to identify novel therapeutic targets.

Chemotherapy and radiation advances: Studies are exploring new combinations of chemotherapy drugs, radiation therapy techniques, and treatment schedules to improve the effectiveness of these treatments while minimizing side effects.

Prevention strategies: Research into lifestyle modifications, dietary interventions, and chemoprevention agents aims to identify strategies for reducing the risk of colorectal cancer.

Health disparities: Efforts are being made to address health disparities in colorectal cancer outcomes, including disparities related to race, ethnicity, socioeconomic status, and geographic location.

Survivorship and quality of life: Research is focusing on improving the long-term quality of life for colorectal cancer survivors through survivorship care plans, psychosocial support, and interventions to manage treatment-related side effects.

Clinical trials: Participation in clinical trials is essential for advancing colorectal cancer research and testing new treatments. Ongoing efforts aim to increase awareness of and access to clinical trials.

Surgical procedure	**No. of patients**	**% of patients**
Abdominoperineal resection	44	20.65%
Rectosigmoidian resection with ileostomy	34	15.96%
Rectosigmoidian resection without ileostomy	96	45.07%
Hartmann procedure	39	18.30%

Table 1.
Surgical procedure and number of patient.

DOI: http://dx.doi.org/10.5772/intechopen.1003904

Patient-centered care: Future research will continue to emphasize patient-centered care, including shared decision-making, supportive care, and addressing the physical and emotional needs of patients and their families.

My retrospective observational study for 5 years between 2014 and 2019 about pelvic recurrence after surgical treatment of rectal cancer is as follows: 219 patients from three surgical centers in Romania, among which 213 of them were treated surgically in three surgical centers in Romania and three of them underwent procedures for treatment of rectal cancer: 39 patients—anterior resection with Hartmann's procedure, 130 patients—anterior resection of rectosigmoid with colorectal anastomosis, and 44 patients—abdominoperineal resection, follow-up for 2 years and pelvic recurrence reported in 19 patients, of whom two patients were shown to have anastomosis recurrence and the highest recurrence rate was reported after Hartmann's procedure. Patients underwent postoperative follow-up for at least 2 years (at 1 month, 3 months, 6 months, 1 year, and 2 years), consisting of anamnesis,;clinical examination; abdominal and pelvic ultrasound; chest radiography; colonoscopy, ultrasound (U/S), CT scan, and MRI (**Table 1**).

Author details

Al Aloul Adnan[1,2*] and Varlas Valentin[3,4]

1 Department of Surgery, Ramnicu Sarat County Hospital, Buzau, Romania

2 Faculty of Nursing Buzau, Biotera University, Romania

3 Filantropia Hospital Clinic, Bucharest, Romania

4 UMF Carol Davila, Bucharest, Romania

*Address all correspondence to: adnanalaloul@yahoo.com

References

[1] Paulus J. Colorectal cancer facts and figures 2020-2022, Amfile///C/Users/Ali/Downloads/introduction (2).docxerican. Cancer Society. 2020;**66**(11):1-9

[2] Bray F, Ferlay J, Soerjomataram I, Siegel RL, Torre LA, Jemal A. Global cancer statistics 2018: GLOBOCAN estimates of incidence and mortality worldwide for 36 cancers in 185 countries, CA. Cancer Journal for Clinicians. 2018;**68**(6):394-424

[3] Center MM, Jemal A, Ward E. International trends in colorectal cancer incidence rates. Cancer Epidemiology, Biomarkers & Prevention. 2009;**18**(6):1688-1694

[4] Glimelius B et al. Cancerul colorectal-Ghid pentru pacienţi-Informaţii bazate pe Ghidurile de Practică Clinică ESMO. Cancerul Color. pentru pacienţi. 2015;**1**:3-6

[5] Angelescu N. Tratat de patologie chirurgicala. Bucharest, Romania: Editura Medicală; 2003

[6] Chow HS, Tilney P, Paraskeva S, Jeyarajah EZ, Purkayastha S. The morbidity surrounding reversal of defunctioning ileostomies: A systematic review of 48 studies including 6,107 cases. International Journal of Colorectal Disease. 2009;**24**(6):711-723

[7] Sauer R et al. Preoperative versus postoperative chemoradiotherapy for rectal cancer. The New England Journal of Medicine. 2004;**351**(17):1731-1740

[8] Mahipal, Grothey A. Role of biologics in first-line treatment of colorectal cancer. Journal of Oncology Practice/American Society of Clinical Oncology. 2016;**12**(12):1219-1228

[9] Pătraşcu TR, Doran H, Musat O. Protezarea anastomozelor colo- rectale cu tub transanal. Chirurgia (Bucur). 2004;**1**(1):99

[10] Ross et al. Recurrence and survival after surgical management of rectal cancer. American Journal of Surgery. 1999;**177**(5):392-395

[11] Bipat S, Glas AS, Slors FJM, Zwinderman AH, Bossuyt PMM, Stoker J. Rectal cancer: Local staging and assessment of lymph node involvement with endoluminal US, CT, and MR imaging - A meta-analysis. Radiology. 2004;**232**(3):773-783

[12] Williams NS, Dixon MF, Johnston D. Reappraisal of the 5 centimetre rule of distal excision for carcinoma of the rectum: A study of distal intramural spread and of patients' survival. The British Journal of Surgery. 1983;**70**(3):150-154

[13] Kwok SPY, Lau WY, Leung KL, Liew CT, Li AKC. Prospective analysis of the distal margin of clearance in anterior resection for rectal carcinoma. The British Journal of Surgery. 1996;**83**(7):969-972

[14] Shirouzu K, Isomoto H, Kakegawa T. Distal spread of rectal cancer and optimal distal margin of resection for sphincter-preserving surgery. Cancer. 1995;**76**(3):388-392

[15] Breugom J et al. Adjuvant chemotherapy after preoperative (chemo) radiotherapy and surgery for patients with rectal cancer: A systematic review and meta-analysis of individual patient data. The Lancet Oncology. 2015;**16**(2):200-207

[16] Kim JC et al. Source of errors in the evaluation of early rectal cancer

by endoluminal ultrasonography. Diseases of the Colon and Rectum. 2001;**44**(9):1302-1309

[17] Li JCM et al. The learning curve for endorectal ultrasonography in rectal cancer staging. Surgical Endoscopy. 2010;**24**(12):3054-3059

[18] Morris OJ, Draganic B, Smith S. Does a learning curve exist in endorectal two-dimensional ultrasound accuracy? Techniques in Coloproctology. 2011;**15**(3):301-311

Chapter 3

On 5G, 6G, mmWave Usage in Colonoscopy

Kumud S. Altmayer

Abstract

For reliable communication, binary hypothesis testing is important to find the error probability. The interest has been growing in short and medium blocklengths also called short packets to implement in the modern day wireless communication system. The colonoscopy diagnosis now uses mmWave which is 5G and 6G. This is utilised for design models to enhance the image technology in the diagnosis of colonoscopy, and endoscopy to facilitate medical practitioners. There is a possibility to use these techniques in medical equipment for real-time support to physicians and operator-independent prediction. The 5G and eventually 6G would enable the expansion to faster processing of data analysis and medical imaging technology.

Keywords: colonoscopy, endoscopy, computational intelligence, histology, noisy channels, 5G, 6G, mmWave, real-time analysis

1. Introduction

The colonoscopy and endoscopy are related to a process of checking the colon. The two are about the internal organs and radiographic visualisation is done by an endoscope. The colonoscopy itself is an endoscopy and it's a nonsurgical procedure. One should note that the visualisation of internal organs is important as far as diagnosis is concerned. Further, it's necessary to make sure nothing extra is developed there and the colon is clean. In this process, a physician will look into it and examine the colon to identify if anything abnormal is growing. Hence, it can be easily cured. As per statistical data, bowel cancer is one of the biggest cancers killers in the United States. The diagnosis done earlier is better to have a proper cure. In the United States, there are several clinics using state-of-the-art technology which is the main topic here. This is where 5G, 6G or mmWave are used which is the latest technology. The usage of equipment and facilities with the latest technology provides a doctor to analyse efficiently in case there are polyps, or other objects showing an abnormal growth in the organ. Colorectal cancer (CRC) may develop in the colon or the rectum as a noncancerous adenomas or polyps over several years. All these precancerous growths can be removed, thus reducing the risk of developing a colon cancer.

This is one of the cancers that is preventable in full if detected, and treated early. The current diagnoses include colonoscopy and upper endoscopy. In general, it's an invasive examination that looks for small growths called polyps within the colon. These procedures are uncomfortable and are in demand. Polyps may not necessarily lead to cancer, but current methods of colonoscopy miss around one (1) in five (5) of them due to old procedures.

The other way to put it is that, there could be a possibility that cancerous polyps are not found despite diagnostic procedures. One of the good places to read a detailed summary about colon cancer, its diagnosis and a procedural treatment will be the web-site of the American Cancer Society and the reference [1].

It has been known that our health-care system is experiencing a tremendous amount of pressure to complete the number of endoscopies required, and also due to the fact that the bowel cancer screening age has been lowered. Further, the appointments were reduced due to the pandemic, now there is a backlog. An individual who is sixty years old or above must take an appointment ahead of time so that he/she gets an opportunity to take care of the endoscopy procedure. The recommendation by the Department of Health and Human Services is the age of sixty and above including the screening for colorectal cancer would be helpful. The colorectal cancer has two parts, one is colon cancer and the other is rectal cancer. Both are equally important.

Research and development (R & D) are the keys to solving several issues the health-care system has. The health-care providers can offer a better service with a higher quality of care to their patients by making use of the new technology solutions. This may include the community services and/or at home. Nowadays, remote diagnosis is also in place. **Table 1** shows the list of one of the topmost clinics in the United States. One may consider using other local clinics and also ask for a referral.

In other words, it's possible to do home screening for this type of colorectal cancer. The usage of AI (artificial intelligence) assisted colonoscopy polyp detection trial will help doctors to improve the quality of patient care, improve the accuracy of detection rates by capturing the information correctly and eventually reduce errors. This kind of method would significantly improve the patient outcomes when assisted in proper and timely diagnoses. Moreover, it will save time for the endoscopy procedure. As far as the cost is concerned, one must enquire by health-care provider.

On the other hand, many clinics still use the older methodology of manual procedure. For example, colon cancer is detected through colonoscopy procedure that is manual requiring extra attention and time from medical practitioners for accurate detection.

Clinic Name	Rate (%)[a]	Target (%)	Results[b]
Mayo Clinic	100	100	100/100
Cedras-Cinai Clinic	92	100	92/100
UCLA Med	90	100	90/100
NYU Langone	88	100	88/100
Huston Methodist	87.5 8	100	87.5/100
Mount Sinai	87.3	100	87.3/100
NY Colombia-Cornell	86	100	86/100
Cleveland Clinic	85.8	100	85.8/100
North-Western Medical	83.9	100	83.9/100
Stanford Healthcare	82.8	100	82.8/100

[a]*These are the topmost.*
[b]*More Gastronomical clinics are available.*

Table 1.
List of best ten hospitals.

Further, this is a longer way to do the detection and not at all comfortable one for patients including for the doctors and nurses who have to perform the procedure with an old method. The AI (artificial intelligence) assisted and "Ultra-fast, low latency 5G networks will transform the Health-care sector". For example, at Airtel, India they have demonstrated this by conducting first colonoscopy trials. Health-care is one of the most promising use cases for 5G, and they collaborated with Apollo Hospitals, India.

Here in the United States, AWS, HealthNet Global are partnering with clinics and hospitals for the usage of the latest technology. Several clinics are already using the ultra-fast 5G technology. The usage of mmWave which will be even faster is in progress. This would certainly assist the doctor's ability to detect. AI usage has helped to improve physician's accuracy in detecting the chronic illnesses and detecting the growth of cancerous cells if any. Early detection and removal of polyps can easily be avoided so that any extra tumour may not become cancerous.

Mayo Clinic and several other clinics have a patient-centric approach that keeps them on an outlook for technologies that can make the outcomes better. With this new technology, one can develop a battery-free communication system for a wireless video capsule endoscope with potential video streaming at a rate of up to fifteen (15) Mega bits per second. An application of an innovative approach by using back-scatter for implants, and a RADAR approach that can remotely read the information from the deep implants, such as the video capsule endoscope. This is used with a 5G deployed network together with cutting-edge computing. Eventually, it should be capable of transmitting the video data from the capsule to a high-performance computing platform in a secure manner. This provides an end-to-end latency to perform polyp detection and its localisation.

This energy-intensive inference by the use of deep learning neural networks technique for polyp detection and localisation can be done in the edge where control signals are sent back to the pill if being used by a doctor to increase the spatial and temporal resolution of the video. Thus, one obtains high-quality images for further analysis. Please see references [2–4]. The access to near real-time data and the ability to make split-second decisions are critical and important in health-care environments. This important sector has the potential to achieve excellent benefits from 5G and 6G or mmWave advanced technologies when implemented as per the needs of a patient as well as the doctors and nurses. This kind of better communication will certainly produce efficiencies in the health-care sector. Diagnostics should be done faster at a fast pace to save time in the diagnosis and treatment of a patient. Transfers of massive files, images and other content will benefit from low latency for fast data transfer. The computer power embedded with 5G and beyond will help to accelerate benefits as we progress with the usage of the latest technology in health-care system. The reader is referred to [3, 5, 6].

We describe the method of artificial neural network simulation for a given dataset, [7] and the results obtained with respect to the survival rate. The simulation results can be compared with [2, 3, 5, 6, 8]. This is the part of machine learning and in part known as deep learning. This is also known as AI (artificial intelligence) assisted program for health-care systems.

2. Colonoscopy and endoscopy methodology

The rapid growth of technology usage in research changes and with the AI-assisted research shows promising results. One needs testing of AI models for a complex system and diagnosis of colonoscopy and endoscopy. The result is acceptable with the analysis of training and testing in this work. This is one of the techniques of deep learning and machine learning.

For histology, it should be mentioned that instead of data, one can use images and work with them to do the deep learning analysis. Digital imaging technology also belongs to 5G, 6G and is of utmost importance to physicians. Thus providing operator-independent pathology prediction. With machine learning and deep learning techniques, one can develop an algorithm as in [2, 5, 9].

2.1 Simulation results

The simulation results are obtained by using the data-set mentioned in the previous section for the analysis of colorectal cancer in males and females. Males may have some form of colon cancer on the right while females may have it on the left of the colon.

Figure 1 shows the results of the rate of survival and frequency of survival.

Figure 2 shows the results of the training of output and the target values. In this figure, the results indicate that each training epoch uses a shaded background. An epoch is a full pass through the entire data-set. It shows that there are nine males on the left and one female on the right. The validation frequency is approximately 87 percent.

2.2 Data-set used

In this study, we are using data-set from Kaggle's web-site for colorectal cancer which was published in 2021. The data-set can be accessed from the reference list [7]. The data-set describes about male, female real colorectal cancer, for health and cancer

Average of DFS (in months)	**Gender**			
Dukes Stage	**Female**	**Male**	**(blank)**	**Grand Total**
A	34	54.53846154		50.6875
C	61	34.5625		39.85
B	29	43.33333333		38.21428571
D	55.5	33.6		37.25
(blank)				
Grand Total	**43**	**41.41666667**		**41.77419355**

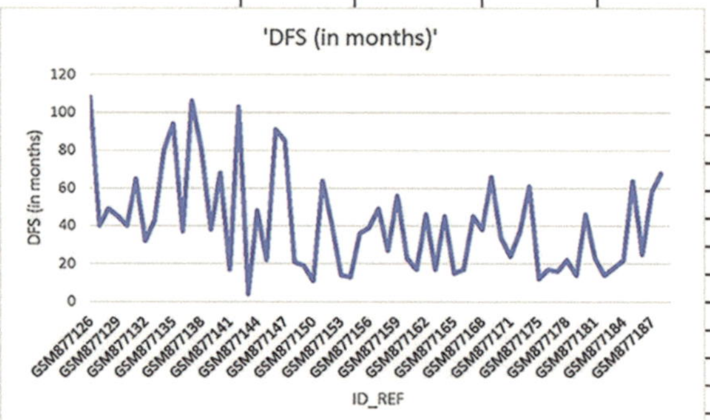

Figure 1.
Average male female DFS.

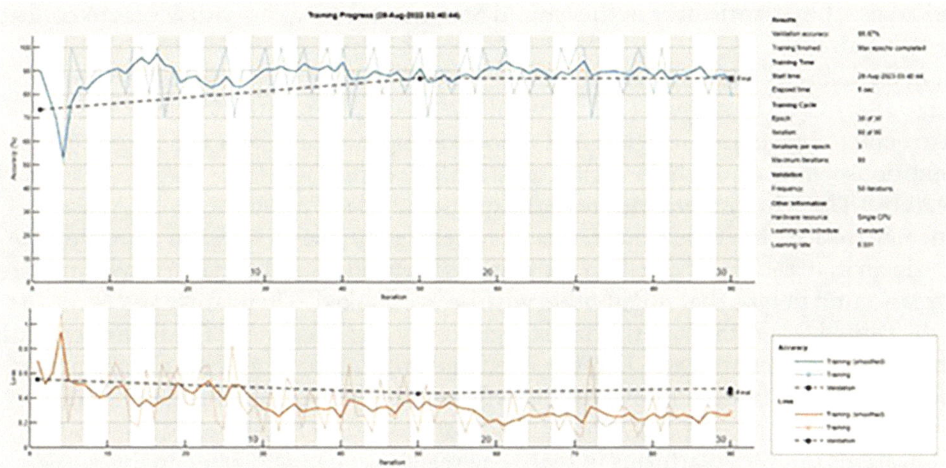

Figure 2.
Validation result.

data analysis. Their analysis is based on probability and histogram charts. Here it's done using MATLAB's method of training and testing model. They also have other data-set that can analyse histology by doing the training and testing model of deep learning with MATLAB toolbox or by using Python language. Please see the references [3–6, 9].

3. Remote technology in colonoscopy and endoscopy

By the use of 5G and remote technology, an innovative new pilot scheme has been launched in the United Kingdom as well as here in the United States at the Mayo Clinic and several other clinics. West Midlands aims to give patients the ability to undergo a procedure to detect the causes of digestive or stomach complaints in the privacy of their homes. Please see **Table 1** for the list of top ten (10) clinics.

Patients awaiting an endoscopy (a procedure whereby a camera is fed into the bowel through a thin tube to detect signs of issues such as cancer) will soon be able to undertake a similar, less invasive procedure from the comfort of their own homes. It's a matter of time before the 5G capability will provide changes to future usage of AI (artificial intelligence).

Further, 6G or mmWave technology will improve with ultra-high speed and low latency in helping clinicians, and medical practitioners to analyse the data, images and video footage recorded. Hence, it will be even quicker identification of polyps, the precursors to cancer and other irregularities, than currently possible.

3.1 An example of AI technology

This is where the MK5G project can be inserted. The MK5G: Connecting Communities Test-bed is leading in the United Kingdom as well as here in the United States in demonstrating how applications of 5G technology can be implemented in a real-world setting. This in turn will improve services within the health-care system. The MK5G project aims to raise the bar for standards of health-care across the Europe and across the Atlantic here in the United States in urban areas with access to connectivity required.

In the United States, researchers at the Mayo Clinic have been investigating the usage of artificial intelligence which would increase polyp detection. In general, gastroenterologists are engaging AI as a tool to improve care for a wide range of health conditions which would help to find elusive signs earlier when the diseases are easily treatable. Thus, in turn will improve the quality of life of a patient. With AI assistance, in the case of colon cancer, the AI system is capable of working alongside the physician in real-time. It can scan the colonoscopy video feed and can draw small, red boxes around polyps that might otherwise be overlooked. There are many clinics here in the United States that use this latest technology of AI-assisted. The invention of this technology enables an "extra helping hand and an extra pair of eyes" for physicians, and staff. This helps to improve the detection rate of polyps, thus saving lives and vastly improving patient care. The data was processed by Avesha edge inferencing applications on AWS platforms in real-time resulting in much faster analysis, the company said in a statement.

Magnetically controlled capsule endoscopy (MCE), with equally favourable diagnostic accuracy as conventional gastroscopy, has become an efficient and comfortable diagnostic modality for GI (gastrointestinal) diseases. An endoscopist could control the movement of the capsule inside the human body precisely through the manipulation of the magnetic robot arm. The non-invasive capsule endoscope, which allows image acquisition after being swallowed, works separately from the control parts of the MCE system. The separable and robotic characteristics of the MCE system provide the technical foundation for remote operation. Moreover, the recent development of the fifth generation of wireless systems (5G), with its high speed, low latency and wide bandwidth, has further supported real-time tele-medicine with reliable networks.

Some real-time remote examinations and surgeries, such as tele-ultrasound, telerobotic spinal surgery and laparoscopic tele-surgery, have been explored and successfully carried out. A 5G-based remote MCE system is such that the remote endoscopist can directly perform the MCE examination on the patient through a remote-control system and the application of a 5G network. This study aimed to evaluate the feasibility and safety of the 5G-based remote MCE system. Communications solutions provider Bharti Airtel and Apollo Hospitals have carried out India's first 5G-driven, artificial intelligence (AI) guided colonoscopy trials. Please see references [2, 9, 10]. Similar work has been done at the Mayo Clinic and several other topmost clinics, and hospitals here in the United States.

In general, as per current protocol, colon cancer is to be detected through a colonoscopy method which is manual and painful. Moreover, patients are reluctant to go through such a procedure. This procedure is performed using a device comprising a light, and flexible tube with light, camera and tools at one end, which are used to extract samples to identify an infected polyp. This method is long, and is discomforting for patients including the doctors and nurses who should perform this procedure which takes around 30 to 40 minutes per case. So, a change with the usage of new technology is helpful and it's becoming available now.

With the new technology of AI-guided colonoscopy procedure, the image processing happens in real-time without any lag even when the physician moves the scope through the colon for it to be overlaid on top of the right element of the colon. In other words, the advent of this technology enables a physician to improve the detection rate of polyps, significantly improving the patient care. An AI-assisted colonoscopy polyp detection trial will be helpful for doctors to improve the quality of patient care, improve the accuracy of detection rates by capturing the information correctly and reduce the error probability.

3.1.1 New technology wins real-time

The capsule endoscopy is considered to be a very safe method for gastrointestinal tract examination. The capsule is mainly excreted with a patient's faeces within 24–48 hours after ingestion. There has been a report of retention of the capsule lasting almost four and a half years although the patient was asymptomatic and did not feel well. However, the risk of bowel obstruction may be countered by an abdominal X-ray to locate the device for removal by endoscopy or surgery. Laser surgery is also an option.

With the introduction of the NaviCam® Stomach Capsule System, an advanced technology has been introduced. This combines the magnetic control with innovative and intelligent software to give medical practitioners external robotic control of the capsule inside the human body. One should know that it's a safe procedure with no extra surgery needed. This is one of the minimally invasive procedures by the use of NaviCam®. This system is guided into real-time with several dimensions (two rotational and three translational planes) by an operator from either making use of a control console or a remote console. Thus, multi-centre blinded study, the NaviCam® Stomach System is considered to be a safe method of visualising the gastric mucosa by the usage of remote magnetic manipulation and it would not require any more need for intubation or sedation (**Table 2**).

The NaviCam® Stomach System can be used in clinics and hospitals both, including the ER (Emergency Room) setting. The ANN (artificial neural network) and CNN (convolutional neural network) diagnostic program systems have shown a good performance in diagnosing gastric focal lesions in MCE (Magnetically controlled capsule endoscopy) images. For the full article, please refer to [2, 5–8].

3.1.2 Data table for the figure used to analyse male female survival rate

Table 2 shows the rate of survival of colon cancer patients. Both males and females are considered. This table shows the results obtained via simulation of the data by using the method of ANN (artificial neural network). This provides a training output

Average DFS	Female(%)[a]	Male (%)	Grand Total[b]
Stage A	34	54.54	50.68
Stage C	61	34.56	39.85
State B	29	43.33	38.21
Data D		100	70/100
Total			41.77/

[a]*The A, B, C and D denote Duke Stages.*
[b]*Last column shows the grand total survival rate.*

Table 2.
Survival data table.

and the target intended to obtain the best results possible to compare the male and female patients who survived the colon cancer.

3.1.3 Ten best clinics for colonoscopy and gastronomy in the United States

In **Table 1**, the top ten best clinics and hospital lists are provided here in the United States. The ranking is calculated using percent calculation in terms of the performance of the clinics and hospitals. There are at least ten more excellent clinics. One may find if searched via the internet by using reference [1]. For example, John Hopkins University medical centre is one of the best clinics as well. It depends to whom a patient believes in. Even a small-town clinic may provide a good diagnosis. Obviously, they may not have the latest technology of AI usage.

4. Conclusions

We provide simulation results by using ANN (artificial neural network) by training and testing methodology including the review of the similar work as shown in [2, 3, 5, 9, 11].

It is to be noted that the number of colorectal cancer cases in the United States has been decreasing since the mid-1980s. During the 2000s, incidence rates dropped from three percent to four percent each year. This was due to increased screening in adults aged 50 and older. From 2011 to 2019, incidence rates continued to decrease by one percent annually. However, incidence has been rising by one percent to two percent each year in younger people since the mid-1990s. It is estimated that the colorectal cancer is one of the fourth most commonly diagnosed cancer in the United States among men and women aged 30 to 39. This gives an idea that there is a need for new technology implementation and diagnostic treatment for CRC.

If proven, the 5G and beyond which is 6G or mmWave capability could one day be paired with AI technologies to help clinicians to analyse the images, video footage and video recorded. This in turn would mean even faster identification of polyps, in comparison to currently possible through manual review.

Clinical Robotic and /or tele-surgery (or remote surgery) is aimed at providing high-quality health-care in the most complex medical interventions and surgeries. Highly-qualified medical expertise will be transferred from the major hospitals to the decentralised ones with the use of remote-surgery, remote diagnostics and tele-medicine resulting in significant cost reduction, and improved efficiency in health-care services. Please read the web-site of clinics that have these options or visit the web-site of the American Cancer Society and reference [1] and also at the topmost clinic list from **Table 1**.

Tele-surgery, where parts of the procedure are controlled by a surgeon from a central site to a remote location, is the most demanding application among the remote health-care services and thus by successfully validating this application, the validation of technology for the entire range of less demanding remote health-care applications that can be implied.

Before 5G, only a few tele-surgeries were carried out and reported by the use of a 4G network. Otherwise, mostly internet and satellite networks were previously used for tele-surgery. A robotic tele-surgery was performed to complete a pituitary tumour resection on a simulated model over the internet with a bandwidth of 1 Giga byte per second in 2015. One can visit to see which clinic or hospital did this kind of surgery at reference [1]. Further, a robotic tele-surgery was performed in the left internal mammary artery dissection in pigs through a satellite network with a maximum bandwidth of 10 Mega bytes per second.

The integration of human and machine generated data will radically change health-care services. Please see the latest data-set at reference [7]. In order to accommodate these health-care needs, an entire communication infrastructure integrating the IoT (internet of things) repositories, AI, super-computing, innovative computational algorithms and edge computing micro-sensors would be needed. This will include processing at the point of data acquisition.

Hence, it will be required to construct or create a "telecommunication ecosystem", which will not only be able to archive, monitor and optimise current activities, but also be used to estimate future trends in the personalised medicine, together with an overall health-care services.

At the moment there are research projects investigating such potential systems that are being implemented on an experimental basis. In the forthcoming future, there is a possibility that the bathroom may also become extensively populated with all types of sensors for automatically monitoring health status, and providing a complete physical examination to update health status on a daily basis, while the person is simply performing the normal daily bathroom activities.

Acknowledgements

The author acknowledges her thanks to In-tech-Open for providing an opportunity to write a book chapter on the modern usage of colonoscopy treatment.

Conflict of interest

The author declares no conflict of interest.

Appendices, addenda and nomenclature

In the subsection, appendix A, a flow chart provides a good idea about the process of colorectal cancer treatment. A figure is also added there and it has been obtained from the web-site called Figure-Fit. Besides that, a short video link will be provided for this chapter on colonoscopy with the latest technology usage as mentioned in this subsection at the end.

Abbreviation and nomenclature

Adenomatous	Polyposis Coli (APC)] A multi-functional tumour suppressor gene. Mutations in this gene are responsible for familial adenomatous polyposis and contributes to many sporadic colorectal cancers.
Bowel cancer	Cancer of the large bowel; also known as colorectal cancer, colon cancer or rectal cancer.

Colon	Part of the large intestine that extends from the end of the small intestine (cecum) to the rectum.
Colonoscope	Flexible, elongated tube that can be inserted through the anus and passed through the colon allowing visualisation of the inside.
Colonoscopy	Visual examination of the inner surface of the colon by means of a colonoscope
Colostomy	Procedure to create an opening of the colon through the skin of the abdomen to allow for the passage of faeces; also, the opening itself.
CLE	An endoscopy procedure that uses a specialised endoscope capable of visualising the mucosal layer of the colon at very high magnification.
CT Graphy	Also known as virtual colonoscopy, a medical imaging procedure that uses low dose radiation computerised tomography (CT) scanning to obtain an interior view of the colon (the large bowel) that is otherwise only seen with a more invasive procedure such as colonoscopy where an endoscope is inserted into the rectum and passed through the entire colon.
ABS	Artificial bowel sphincter
ANN	Artificial Neural Network
CI	Confidence Interval
CNN	Convolutional Neural Network
CISNET	Cancer Intervention and Surveillance Modelling Network
COCOS	Colonoscopy or Colonography for Screening
C-RADS	Colonography Reporting and Data System
CRC	Colorectal cancer
CRC-SPIN	Colorectal Cancer Simulated Population Model for Incidence and Natural History
CT	Computed tomography
DFS	Disease-Free Survival
ESGAR	European Society of Gastrointestinal and Abdominal Radiology
DNN	Deep Neural Network
GI	Gastrointestinal
MAP-2	Microtubule-associated protein 2
NORCCAP	Norwegian Colorectal Cancer Prevention
PDT	Population doubling time
SCORE	Screening for Colon and Rectum
SBO	Small bowel obstruction
SPS	Serrated polyposis syndrome

Appendix A

In this work, we have analysed the colorectal cancer by using an artificial neural network with a data-set obtained from Kaggle's web-site. A flowchart is being added that shows a basic idea of colonoscopy treatment with 5G, 6G or mmWave technology.

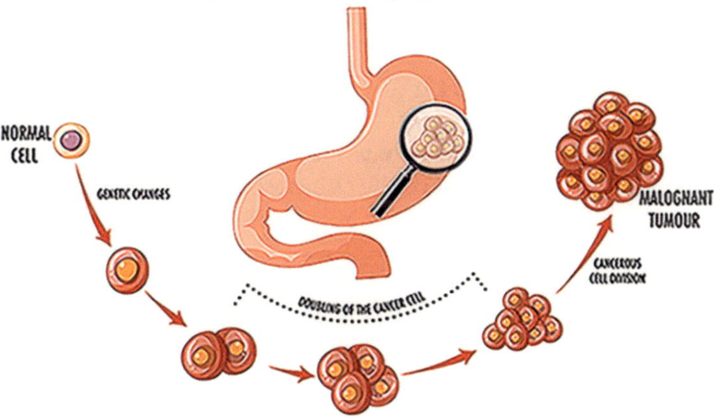

Figure 3.
Colon cancer development.

Figure 3 shows the development of colon cancer. This figure was obtained from https://www.freepik.com/free-photos-vectors/colorectal-cancer.

The next **Figure 4** in the form of a flowchart also shows how the colon cancer develops and can be treated.

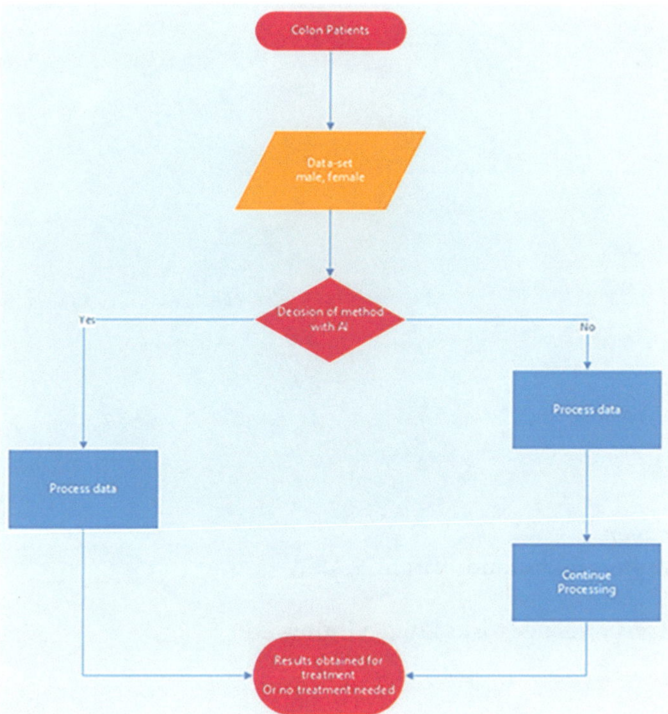

Figure 4.
Colon cancer development, treatment.

Video materials

A video of this chapter is submitted separately. It will be featured as a link inside the text as ColonmmWaveKSA.mp4 which does exceed to 100 MB of limit. The video link will be placed in Appendix A.

Link: https://youtu.be/Wg5uSo4AtVs

Filename: ColonmmWaveKSA.mp4.

The citations are the same which are listed in the references.

The Caption: A short explanation of the colonoscopy treatment with 5G, 6 g and mmWaves.

Author details

Kumud S. Altmayer
Independent Author, Richmond, Virginia, USA

*Address all correspondence to: ksa2te@virginia.edu

References

[1] Available from: https://www.https://www.cancer.net/navigating-cancer-care/diagnosing-cancer/tests-and-procedures/types-endoscopy [Accessed: 2023]

[2] Yang T, NingLiang JL, Young Y, Li Y, Huang Q, Li R, et al. Intelligent imagining Technology in Diagnosis of colorectal cancer using deep learning. Journal IEEE Access. 2019;**7**:178839-178847. DOI: 10.1109/ACCESS.2019.2958124. [Accessed: December 23, 2019]

[3] Kather J, Weis CA, Bianconi F, et al. Multi-class texture analysis in colorectal cancer histology. Scientific Reports. 2016;**6**:27988. DOI: 10.1038/srep27988

[4] Georgiou KE, Georgiou E, Satava RM. 5G use in healthcare: The future is present. JSLS. 2021;**25**(4):e2021.00064. DOI: 10.4293/JSLS.2021.00064. PMID: 35087266; PMCID: PMC8764898

[5] Yang T, NingLiang JL, Young Y, Li Y, Huang Q, Li R, et al. 5G-based RemotColorectal cancer facts figures 2020-2022e magnetically controlled capsule endoscopy for examination of the stomach and small bowel. United European Gastroenterology Journal. 2022;**11**. DOI: 10.1002/ueg2.12339. [Accessed: 13 October 2022]

[6] Colorectal Cancer Facts & Figures 2020-2022. Available from: https://www.cancer.org/content/dam/cancer-org/research/cancer-facts-and-statistics/colorectal-cancer-facts-and-figures/colorectal-cancer-facts-and-figures-2020-2022.pdf [Accessed: November 04, 2016]

[7] Available from: https://www.kaggle.com/datasets/amandam1/colorectal-cancer-patients [Accessed: November 2021]

[8] Morgado-Diaz JA, editor. Gastrointestinal Cancers. Brisbane, Australia: Exon Publications; Baojun Duan, Yaning Zhao et al, Chapter 1. Available from: https://www.ncbi.nlm.nih.gov/books/NBK586003. [Accessed: September 30, 2022]

[9] Mahmood S, Ghazel T, Khan M, Zubair M, Naseem M, Faiz T, et al. Malignancy detection in lung and colon Histopathalogy Imgaes using transfer learning with class selective image processing. Journal IEEE Access. 2022;**10**:25657-25668. DOI: 10.1109/ACCESS.2022.3150924. [Accessed: March 10, 2022]

[10] Airtel, Apollo, AWS conduct India's first 5G-driven, AI-guided colonoscopy trial. Available from: https://www.teleinfotoday.com/press-releases/airtel-apollo-aws-conduct-indias-first-5g-driven-ai-guided-colonoscopy-trial [Accessed: July 26, 2023]

[11] Waye JD, Rex DK, Williams CB, editors. Colonoscopy: Principles and Practice. Wiley-Blackwell. 2nd edition. 2009. [Accessed: 2003]. ISBN: 978-1-405-17599-9

Chapter 4

Colonoscopy, Barriers, and Challenges for Colorectal Cancer Screening in Developing Countries

Arum Linangkung

Abstract

Colorectal cancer (CRC) is the third most common cancer worldwide. The incidence of CRC is rising in developing countries but decreasing in developed countries due to the widespread use of screening and surveillance colonoscopy. The implementation of screening and surveillance programs remains a challenge in developing countries, especially Indonesia. Increasing screening rates among underserved populations in Indonesia, the world's fourth most populous country, will reduce the global burden of colorectal cancer. The need for an integrated screening program in its healthcare system will provide a successful screening program. The purpose of a screening colonoscopy is to reveal the asymptomatic population with a certain disease through the use of an effective investigation to detect and treat the disease before it advances. Screening improves the prognosis of patients and the mortality rate. Removal of neoplastic polyps such as adenomas, the precancerous lesions during colonoscopy, is the cornerstone of screening colonoscopy. The detection rate is a measure of screening colonoscopy performance quality. Technology has been used to improve detection, such as mechanical technology (Endocuff) and optical, such as magnification, endocytoscopy, virtual chromoendoscopy, and recently artificial intelligence. Indonesia is a nation that is significantly affected by CRC and will benefit from screening colonoscopy.

Keywords: colonoscopy, colorectal cancer, developing country, screening, barrier

1. Introduction

Colorectal cancer is the most common type of gastrointestinal malignancy, the third most diagnosed cancer worldwide, and the second most common cause of cancer death. Among other continents, according to GLOBOCAN 2020 reports, Asia has the highest prevalence of 50%. Of these, 75% of cases are reported in East Asia. Indonesia has the highest estimated number of new cases (32%; 34.189 cases), followed by Thailand. The incidence of colorectal cancer in Indonesia is 12.8 per 100,000 citizens, with a mortality rate of 9.5% from all malignancies. This high incidence ranked Indonesia, the top third in the world [1].

Identification of the population at risk and screening of asymptomatic patients is therefore crucial imperatives. Most colorectal cancer is slow-growing, arising from precancerous lesions such as adenomatous polyps or sessile serrated lesions. This slow growth gives a window of time to screen for both early cancer and precancer lesions. If colorectal cancer is diagnosed at an early stage, however, it is one of the most curable malignancies.

Considering the increasing number of locally advanced and advanced cases of colorectal cancer in developing countries, there is an urgent need to implement screening strategies. Screening programs are aimed at early detection, recognizing early signs and symptoms of the presence of the disease, and treating patients with curative intent. Colonoscopy, as step two of screening, has been proven to improve the prognosis and lower the mortality rate. Therefore, in order to maximize the benefits of cancer prevention programs, it is worth identifying, and defining investment opportunities for colonoscopy in the healthcare system, especially in populous developing countries like Indonesia.

Global differences are reported in colonoscopy implementation in developing countries. It is likely due to differences and limitations in access to diagnostic and treatment facilities in most developing countries, a lack of resources for the health care system and cancer care is commonly seen. There are social, cultural, and structural ranging from poverty, limited access, the misbelief of the incurability of any tumor, the fear of stigma, and sociodemographic barriers related to proper health facility accessibility due to long distances or unaffordable cancer services not covered by national health insurance [2].

Colonoscopy is highly sensitive and specific for colorectal cancer detection and polyp removal. This invasive and resourceful procedure is performed in more developed countries in organized mass screening protocols in persons with a positive response to a filter fecal occult blood test (FOBT). However, compliance is still limited, cost is high, and complications can occur. In recent years, colonoscopy tends to be performed more often as a primary test in opportunistic nonorganized screening for asymptomatic persons asking for prevention.

In developing countries, the risk of colorectal cancer may increase, contrasting with a persistent weakness in organized mass screening under the control of Health Authorities. The discrepancy should encourage the growth of opportunistic indications for primary colonoscopy in spite of its high cost. However, this is not a population-based strategy of prevention. Hence, the prognosis, mortality rate, and burden of disease have improved through the implementation of effective screening.

The advantages of colonoscopy are both its benefit of simultaneous diagnostic and therapeutic procedures. Its direct visualization and marking site option are very useful in the era of multimodality optimal cancer care via personalized medicine. It assists surgeons in deciding on a tailored surgery approach and the possibility of the option of chemoradiation modalities.

Disadvantages of colonoscopy are its invasiveness, risk of complications (such as perforation and hemorrhage), the need for bowel preparation, and its burden on resources and associated costs. Colonoscopy detects and visualizes directly the structural identification of many diminutive small adenomatous and sessile serrated polyps.

2. The role of the essential triangle factor in screening colonoscopy

Colonoscopy is the gold standard procedure for the early detection of colorectal cancer and premalignant adenomatous polyps. Screening procedures can be indicated in two conditions: a primary colonoscopy or a secondary colonoscopy. The primary colonoscopy was conducted without a filter test in nonorganized or opportunistic screening of the average risk person group, aged 50 years or more. The secondary colonoscopy was the stage two program after a positive first stage filter of fecal occult blood test (FOBT) in an organized mass screening protocol by Health Authorities in a population of asymptomatic persons of both sexes in age 50 to 70 years.

The colonoscopy screening program will be effective and successful through a solid collaboration between the essential triangle factors that consist of the role of Health Authorities, compliance of population or patient adherence, and lastly, the provider side (**Figure 1**).

2.1 National Health Policy

The policy of prevention deserves to be generalized in developing countries. Government support, public health campaigns, and nationwide strategies must be formulated as the authority's priority. In each country, cancer prevention is under the control of a National Health Service of the Ministry of Health, like in Indonesia [3]. The National Authorities actively encourage the control of environmental carcinogenic factors linked to diet with excess calories and lack of vegetables and physical activity. The organization of a screening policy of secondary prevention depends on the Colorectal Cancer National Guideline. Developing countries with low resources tend to concentrate resources on treatment services in their National Health Care System. Emerging countries with higher resources have already built better healthcare structures [4]. In Indonesia, colonoscopy as a step two screening procedure has been established in the national colorectal cancer control guideline, but heterogeneity persists in rural and urban areas. An integrated national registry will help to scale up and enable the identification of discrepancies, false-negative cases, and interval cancers. National reporting systems of screening activate better monitoring consistency as well as continuous quality assurance and further cancer control planning. Information technology can assist coverage of screening tests by a model of mobile application based on the Asia Pacific Colorectal Screening (APCS) score.

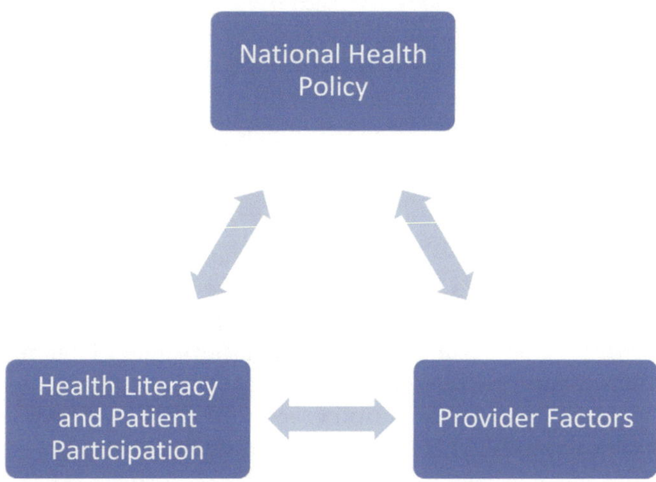

Figure 1.
Essential triangle factors in screening colonoscopy.

2.2 Health literacy and patient participation

Public education and general practitioner insight into the risk factors of colorectal cancer and referral indication need to be pursued. Health promotion increases public and physician awareness and strengthens the compliance of the screened population and patient adherence to cancer surveillance. Physicians in primary health services should not ignore the presence of blood in the stool of patients older than 50 years old as simply hemorrhoids. Investigation into the risk factor must be highlighted, particularly for patients with genetic predispositions in the first degree. Asymptomatic patients at average risk should also be promoted.

Patient selection is still based on primary and secondary procedures. An educated and well-informed population with risk factors for colorectal cancer tends to get the primary colonoscopy as an opportunistic screening. Hence, the secondary procedure is the follow-up intervention after a positive noninvasive screening option, like FOBT screening, has been established in many developing countries [5].

Discrepancy must be avoided as rural areas have more population with a lower education level than urban areas. Geographical issues still exist in many developing countries, such as Indonesia, due to colonoscopy services are commonly in the sub or urban areas, in tertiary hospitals. Some patients need to put more effort into accommodation. Social and community support sometimes helps in some local conditions, especially for those who live in archipelago areas.

The urban area also has its own problem with screening procedures. The change in sedentary lifestyle, smoking, alcohol consumption, "westernized" food, and lack of physical activity resulting in obesity, make the risk of colorectal cancer become higher. The incidence and prevalence of young colorectal cancer patient in developing countries tends to increase recently, projected to continue over the next decade. Screening consideration for the working-class population, in productive age, is getting important. Diagnosing colorectal cancer early is cheaper than treating advanced malignancy. The short and long-term term-productivity loss also could be minimized.

Social media impact by health volunteers, influencers, or public figures promotion will provide an insight that colonoscopy as an invasive procedure is more culturally and psychosocially acceptable.

Successful participant recruitment through the repeating multifactorial cycle results in strong fundamental patient adherence and compliance with colonoscopy screening (**Figure 2**). Each of the cycle factors could be explored particularly in many creative and innovative ways. Continuous activities that engage the public, patients, and primary care physicians should be encouraged, like cancer awareness month, social campaigns, and sports events.

2.3 Provider factors

Financial reimbursement and human resources are the keys on the provider side. Financial limitations in many developing countries are still problematic and require a defining concern and model to fill the gap [6]. Reimbursement from national health insurance or private insurance must promptly accept the need for screening colonoscopy. Delayed procedures due to multilevel administrative referral systems and hierarchical insurance approval may limit compliance and coverage.

Gastroenterologists and digestive surgeons both can perform the procedure effectively. The aim is the patient-oriented goal to achieve early detection of colorectal cancer. Complete colonoscopy units for performing full colonoscopy equipment

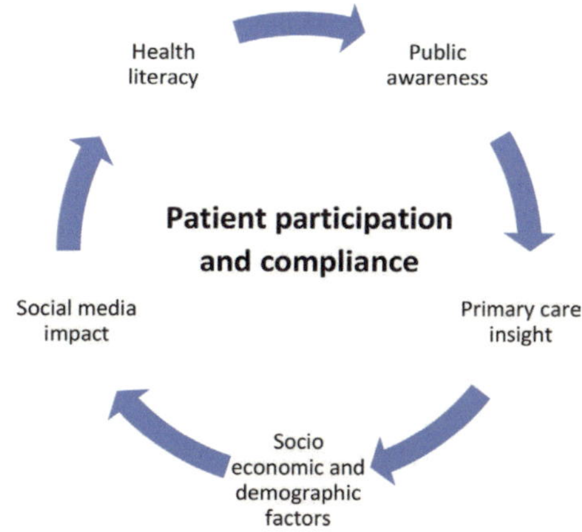

Figure 2.
Patient participation and compliance.

including endoscopes with biopsy puncture facilities and polypectomy snares need to be standardized in every hospital. Personalized colonoscopy plans and additional technology in colonoscopy can be established through partnership training between the developed world and developing countries to build better capacity levels. Advanced technology such as mechanical technology (Endocuff) and optical, such as magnification, endocytoscopy, and virtual chromoendoscopy could be introduced to invite investors. Information technology like artificial intelligence is also required in the near future to assist well-trained operators and junior staff in training in order to improve coverage, safety level, performance quality, detection rate, and treatment rate [7].

Epidemiological research in developing countries and cancer registries helps to picture the landscape of colorectal cancer in a particular area and build patient navigation. The ratio between patient and provider needs to be calculated to avoid a long waiting list for the procedure. A national cost-effective study must be conducted in the developing world in order to analyze the cost-effective colonoscopy screening model and to integrate the research component into the national cancer control plan.

3. Conclusion

Overcoming barriers in the implementation of colonoscopy remains a challenge in developing countries, especially Indonesia. Indonesia, the world's fourth most populous country, is significantly affected by colorectal cancer and will benefit from colonoscopy. Increasing screening uptake among underserved populations in Indonesia should be supported.

As a part of optimal cancer care in developing countries with increasing resources, colonoscopy procedures should be developed its feasibility as a screening measure and integrated policy for colorectal cancer prevention and surveillance. Health Authorities, compliance of the population, and provider resources are the essential triangle factors in colonoscopy sustainability.

In current practice, the opportunities for collaborative service and future research between developing countries and developed countries are widely open and will enhance the availability and detection rate of colonoscopy as the gold standard screening procedure in reducing the global burden of colorectal cancer, with an impact on mortality and survival.

Acknowledgements

The authors gratefully acknowledge the colonoscopy facilities provided by Dr. Suhardi Hardjolukito Central Air Force National Hospital and all its staff in Public Health Services. The authors would specifically like to thank all the faculties and staff of the Digestive Surgery Division of RSUP Dr. Sardjito Hospital Yogyakarta-Indonesia, Digestive Surgery Division of RSUP Dr. Kariadi Hospital Semarang-Indonesia, and the Advanced Surgery Training Center of National University Hospital Singapore for the coordination and opportunity in the context of the advanced colonoscopy training.

Conflict of interest

The authors declare no conflict of interest.

Author details

Arum Linangkung
Division of Digestive Surgery, Department of Surgery, Dr. Suhardi Hardjolukito Central Air Force National Hospital – Academic Hospital of Faculty of Medicine, Public Health and Nursing, Universitas Gadjah Mada, Yogyakarta, Indonesia

*Address all correspondence to: arum.linangkung@gmail.com

References

[1] Sung H, Ferlay J, Siegel RL, et al. Global cancer statistics 2020: GLOBOCAN estimates of incidence and mortality worldwide for 36 cancers in 185 countries. CA: A Cancer Journal for Clinicians. 2021. DOI: 10.3322/caac.21660

[2] Ahmed F. Barriers to colorectal cancer screening in the developing world: The view from Pakistan. World Journal of Gastrointestinal Pharmacology and Therapeutics. 2013;**4**(4):83-85. DOI: 10.4292/wjgpt.v4.i4.83

[3] Komite Penanggulangan Kanker Nasional Departemen Kesehatan Republik Indonesia. Pedoman Nasional Pelayanan Kedokteran Tata Laksana Kanker Kolorektal (National Consensus and Guideline). Jakarta: Kemenkes RI (Ministry of Health Republic of Indonesia); 2018. Available from: https://yankes.kemkes.go.id/unduhan/fileunduhan_1610413859_111090.pdf

[4] Khuhaprema T, Sangrajrang S, Lalitwongsa S, et al. Organised colorectal cancer screening in Lampang Province, Thailand: Preliminary results from a pilot implementation programme. BMJ Open. 2014;**4**:e003671. DOI: 10.1136/bmjopen-2013-003671

[5] Purnomo HD, Permatadewi CO, Prasetyo A, Indiarso D, Hutami HT, Puspasari D, et al. Colorectal cancer screening in Semarang, Indonesia: A multicenter primary health care based study. PLoS One. 2023;**18**(1):e0279570. DOI: 10.1371/journal.pone.0279570

[6] Schliemann D, Ramanathan K, Matovu N, O'Neill C, Kee F, Su TT, et al. The implementation of colorectal cancer screening interventions in low-and middle-income countries: A scoping review. BMC Cancer. 2021;**21**(1):1125. DOI: 10.1186/s12885-021-08809-1

[7] Shaukat A, Levin TR. Current and future colorectal cancer screening strategies. Nature Reviews. Gastroenterology & Hepatology. 2022;**19**:521-531. DOI: 10.1038/s41575-022-00612-y

Chapter 5

Modern Approach in the Management of Malignant Colorectal Polyp

Umid Kumar Shrestha

Abstract

Malignant colorectal polyp refers to the polyp in which the neoplastic lesion invades into but not beyond the submucosa. The morphological features and surface patterns of the malignant polyps are examined by the white-light and image-enhanced endoscopy, which help to predict the depth of invasion of neoplastic lesions. The deep submucosal invasion is associated with a high risk of residual cancer and lymph node metastasis. The image-enhanced endoscopy is useful in identifying the malignant polyp amenable for endoscopic resection or require formal oncological surgery. After the endoscopic resection of the polyp, the thorough histopathological assessment is required to determine the possibility of residual tumor, recurrence, and lymph node involvement. The presence of high-risk features (deep submucosal invasion, poor differentiation, lymphovascular invasion, <1 mm resection margin, piecemeal resection, and tumor budding) indicates a need for surgical resection with lymph node clearance. In low-risk cases, the endoscopic resection is considered adequate and further surveillance is advised. The final decision about the endoscopic resection versus surgical resection of malignant polyp needs to be individualized and should be based not only on polyp related characteristics but also on comorbidities, local resources, expertise availability, and patient's preference.

Keywords: malignant colorectal polyp, submucosal invasion, histological feature, endoscopic resection, surgery

1. Introduction

Malignant colorectal polyp (MP) refers to the polyp in which the cancer cells invade into but not beyond the submucosa, regardless of lymph node involvement [1]. Colorectal cancer (CRC) is defined as the invasion of cancer cells beyond the muscularis mucosa. Since the colonic mucosa is devoid of lymphatics, the cancer cells confined to the muscularis mucosa have a negligible risk for lymph node metastasis (LNM) and hence are defined as benign (non-malignant) polyps [2]. According to the American Joint Committee on Cancer tumor-node metastasis classification system, an MP represents early CRC and is categorized as pT1 [3]. Different studies have shown that at least 0.2–8.3% of colorectal polyps are MPs [4–7]. The CRC has become the third most commonly diagnosed form of cancer, and its incidence reaches approximately 1.9 million cancer cases each year (10% of all new cancer cases globally) [8]. Traditionally, the incidence of CRC increases strongly with age and is highest in Western, affluent countries, but the change in the lifestyle has made its incidence increasing in many less developed countries and in younger generations in both developed and developing countries [8].

The CRC arises from the progressive accumulation of genetic and epigenetic alterations. The adenoma-to-carcinoma sequence in development of CRC is shown in the **Figure 1**. The sequence involves the transformation of normal colorectal epithelium to adenoma and ultimately to invasive and metastatic tumor. Such malignant transformation requires up to 15 years, depending on the characteristics of the lesion and on other independent risk factors, such as gender, body weight, body mass index, physical inactivity [9]. The chromosomal instability (CIN), microsatellite instability (MSI), and CpG island methylator phenotype (CIMP) pathways are responsible for genetic and epigenetic instability in CRC [10, 11]. The CIN pathway consists of activation of proto-oncogene Kirsten-ras (K-ras) located on chromosome 12p and inactivation of at least three tumor suppression genes, namely, loss of APC (Adenomatous Polyposis Coli gene) located on chromosome 5q, DCC (Deleted on Colorectal Cancer gene) located within the region of loss of heterozygosity (LOH) of long arm of chromosome 18q, and p53 located on chromosome 17p [10, 11].

With the increasing CRC screening programs, the detection of early CRC has become possible, leading to an increase in the number of people identified as having MP [12–14]. There is often a dilemma regarding the management of MP: the first dilemma is at the time of colonoscopy, when the endoscopist must decide whether a suspicious polyp can be safely endoscopically resected; the second dilemma is after pathologic examination of a polypectomy specimen, when a decision must be made about attempted endoscopic re-excision, surgical resection, or surveillance. The management decision requires an assessment of the endoscopic and pathological features, risk of adverse outcome after endoscopic polypectomy, risk of surgery, and the available surgical options. There are additional considerations in high-risk patients, for instance, those with a family history suggesting hereditary nonpolyposis colorectal cancer (HNPCC), long-standing inflammatory bowel disease, and familial polyposis. This chapter deals primarily with the average-risk patient with an aim to review the endoscopic and pathological features of MP and to discuss about the management strategies of MP.

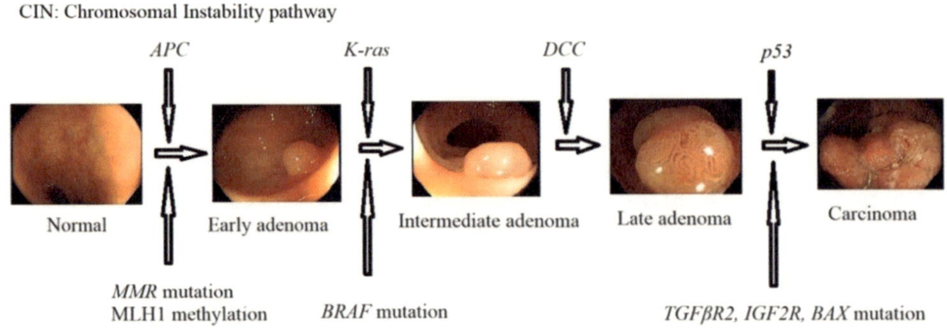

Figure 1.
Adenoma-to-carcinoma sequence in development of colorectal cancer.

2. Endoscopic evaluation

During colonoscopy, all colorectal lesions should be examined by white-light and image-enhanced techniques to differentiate between adenomas and CRC and to predict the depth of invasion [13, 15]. The deep submucosal invasion (SMI) is associated with a high risk of residual cancer and LNM [13, 16]. Gross morphological features and polyp surface patterns are carefully examined during endoscopic evaluation of polyp.

2.1 Gross morphological features

The endoscopic gross features of malignancy include an irregular surface contour, ulceration, firm (or hard) consistency, and broadening of the stalk [17–23]. Although polyps with these features are not invariably malignant, any lesion with malignant characteristics should be carefully evaluated in order to identify the resectable adenoma.

The Paris classification should be used as following for the endoscopic classification of superficial colorectal lesions: polypoid (pedunculated 0-Ip and sessile 0-Is), non-polypoid (elevated 0-IIa, flat 0-IIb, depressed 0-IIc), and excavated or ulcerated lesions (0-III) [16]. The risk of MP (and CRC) seems to be directly proportional to polyp size and the presence of depression: with the risk being as high as 40% in smaller lesions (6–10 mm) to nearly all lesions measuring more than 20 mm [24–26]. The Paris Classification does not address the lateral spreading tumor (LST), which is defined as the superficial non-polypoid colorectal lesion measuring more than 10 mm in diameter, with flat (0-II) or sessile (0-Is) morphology, extending laterally rather than vertically along the colonic wall. On routine colonoscopy, the incidence of LST is approximately 9% [25]. The LST can be broadly subdivided into the granular (LST-G) or non-granular (LST-NG) type [27].

The risk of SMI is as high as 30% in LST-G of more than 30 mm size with mixed-size nodules, whereas LST-G with a homogenous nodular pattern has a low risk of invasion (<2%) [28]. LST-NG is characterized by a smooth surface and can be either flat or pseudo-depressed. The LST-NG with pseudo-depression carries the highest risk of SMI among LSTs (31.6%; 95%CI: 19.8–43.4%) [29].

The location is another important risk factor for SMI. The LST-G mixed type or LST-NG lesion in the rectosigmoid colon carries the highest risk for malignancy [30]. Within the serrated pathway, most carcinomas arise in the cecum or ascending colon, and approximately one-third arise in the rectum [31].

Other gross morphological features that correlate with SMI have also been studied. In one prospective multicenter study including more than 2000 lesions >10 mm, it was found that non-lifting, chicken-skin sign (pale yellow-speckled mucosa), edge retraction, depressed areas, fold convergence, induration, ulceration, and polyp over polyp were all significantly associated with deep SMI [32]. However, the sensitivity of these features for diagnosing deep SMI seems to be low, ranging from 0.18 to 0.68, with specificity varying from 0.8 to 0.98 [33].

2.2 Polyp surface pattern

Besides gross morphology, the risk of SMI can also be assessed by the surface vascular and pit pattern of polyp, which helps in reaching the management decisions. The polyp surface is characterized by image-enhanced endoscopy (IEE), which can be performed by conventional chromoendoscopy and electronic or virtual chromoendoscopy. The conventional chromoendoscopy is dye-based (contrast: indigo carmine; absorptive: crystal violet) and assesses the pit pattern, whereas the electronic or virtual chromoendoscopy is equipment-based (Olympus: NBI; Pentax: I-scan; Fujifilm: BLI, LCI) and assesses the capillary pattern. The polyp surface characterization has been classified by different methods, including Narrow-Band Imaging International Colorectal Endoscopic (NICE) classification system, Japan NBI Expert Team (JNET) classification system, Kudo pit pattern nomenclature, and others.

2.2.1 NICE classification system

Narrow-band imaging (NBI) is a form of electronic or virtual chromoendoscopy initially developed by Sano *et al.* in 1999 [34, 35]. The NBI enables detailed assessment of the capillary mucosal pattern of polyps by filtering white light into specific wavelengths to enhance the superficial microvascular structures [34, 35]. The NBI has been used for the optical diagnosis of colorectal tumors in NICE classification system, which is based on the color, vessels, and surface pattern on endoscopy [36, 37]. In this classification scheme, polyps can be divided into three categories (type 1, 2 or 3) based on their appearance (**Table 1**). NICE type 1 and 2 polyps are benign and can be resected endoscopically. Type 3 polyps are characterized by disrupted/missing vessel pattern and amorphous or absent surface pattern on NBI and are highly suggestive of deep SMI, requiring surgical resection.

2.2.2 JNET classification system

The JNET introduced an NBI-magnifying endoscopic classification system for colorectal polyps in 2014 [36, 38]. The JNET system classifies colorectal polyps into four types (Types 1, 2A, 2B, and 3) (**Table 2**). Type 3 polyps are characterized by irregular or amorphous vessel and surface patterns under magnified endoscopy with NBI; these type 3 polyps are highly suggestive of deep SMI and require surgical resection.

2.2.3 Kudo's pit pattern

Kudo and colleagues classified colorectal polyps according to their appearance, structure, and staining patterns by using magnifying endoscopy [39, 40]. Type I pits appear as roundish pits; type II pits appear as stellar or papillary pits; type III-s pits are small roundish, tubular pits (smaller than type I), and type III-L are roundish and

	Type 1	**Type 2**	**Type 3**
Color	Same or lighter than background	Browner relative to background	Brown to dark brown relative to background
Vessels	None or lacy vessels	Brown vessels	Disrupted or missing vessels
Surface pattern	Dark or white spots of uniform size	Oval, tubular, or branched white structures	Amorphous or absent surface pattern
Most likely pathology	Hyperplastic and sessile serrated polyp	Adenoma	Deep submucosal invasive cancer

Table 1.
NBI International Colorectal Endoscopic (NICE) classification system.

	Type 1	Type 2A	Type 2B	Type 3
Vessel pattern	Invisible	Regular caliber and distribution (meshed/spiral)	Variable caliber, irregular distribution	Loose vessel areas, interruption of thick vessels
Surface pattern	Regular dark or white spots similar to surrounding mucosa	Regular (tubular/branched/papillary)	Irregular or obscure	Amorphous areas
Most likely pathology	Hyperplastic or sessile serrated polyps	Low-grade dysplasia	High grade dysplasia/shallow submucosal invasive cancer	Deep submucosal invasive cancer

Table 2.
Japan Narrow-band imaging Expert Team (JNET) classification system.

tubular pits (larger than type I); type IV pits appear as branch-like or gyrus-like pits, and type V pits appear as amorphous, nonstructured pits [39, 40].

Most colorectal polyps (Kudo pit pattern types I through IV) are benign polyps and are amenable to endoscopic resection, whereas those with Kudo pit pattern V are suggestive of deep SMI and require surgical resection [26, 41].

3. Artificial intelligence

Artificial intelligence (AI) has emerged as an exciting tool in identifying the endoscopic resectability in colorectal polyps by differentiating noninvasive and superficially submucosal invasive neoplasms and deeply invasive cancer. The AI white light systems have shown high accuracy, sensitivity, and specificity in predicting the feasibility of curative endoscopic resection of large colonic lesions [42, 43]. In a study done by Kudo *et al.*, the AI model was validated to identify T1 colorectal tumors at risk for metastasis to the lymph nodes [44]. At this point of time, incorporating AI into clinical practice in the management algorithm of MP may be challenging, but the results of the AI study provide valuable insights into the future trends and potential of AI in the management of MP.

4. Pathologic evaluation

Accurate histopathological assessment is critical in determining adequacy of endoscopic resection of MP, and hence, every effort must be made to retrieve the entire specimen. This is easier for pedunculated polyps than for large sessile polyps that are removed in piecemeal fashion. Saline injection to provide a cushion of normal mucosa under a sessile polyp can greatly aid in the completeness of removal.

4.1 Depth of submucosal invasion (SMI)

The level of SMI is important in predicting the outcome of MP in both pedunculated and sessile polyps. Studies have shown that deeper depth of invasion is related to increased LNM and a poorer outcome [45–47].

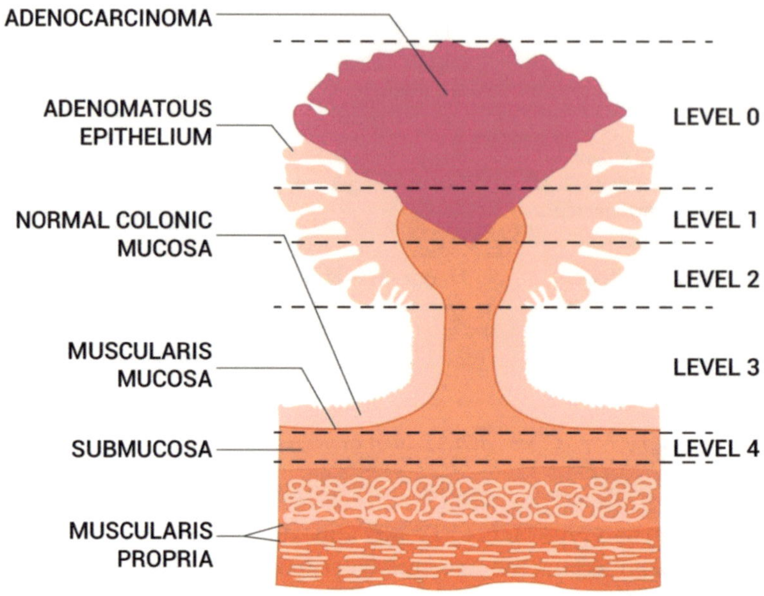

Figure 2.
Haggitt classification system of pedunculated polyp (adapted from Haggitt et al [45]).

The Haggitt classification is used to describe the level of invasion (0—neoplastic cells confined to the mucosa, 1—head, 2—neck, 3—stalk, 4—submucosa of underlying colonic wall) in pedunculated polyps (**Figure 2**) [45]. The study done by Haggitt *et al.* showed that a depth of invasion to Haggitt level 4 was a significant adverse prognostic factor for pedunculated MP. Another study done by Nivatvongs *et al.* showed that there was no incidence of lymph node metastasis for pedunculated Haggitt level 1 to 3, but the risk of lymph node metastasis was as high as 27% for level 4 lesions [48]. For sessile polyps, the Kikuchi classification is used, in which three levels are present based on the degree of SMI: Sm1–invasion into the upper third of the submucosa; Sm2–invasion into the middle third; and Sm3–invasion into the lower third (**Figure 3**) [46]. The study done by Kikuchi *et al.* showed that the risk of metastasis was 0% in Sm1 lesions but increased to as high as 14.4% in Sm3 lesions [46]. Another study done by Kitajima *et al.* showed that for sessile MP, the risk of LNM was 0% if the depth of SMI was less

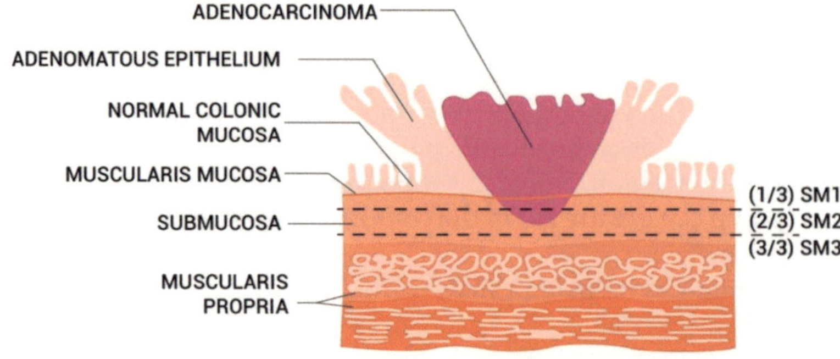

Figure 3.
Kikuchi classification system of sessile polyp (adapted from Kikkuchi et al [46]).

than 1000 μm but increased to more than 11.5% when the depth of invasion exceeded 1000 μm [47]. In a meta-analysis by Beaton *et al.*, it was shown that that the risk of LNM was significantly higher when the depth of SMI was more than 1000 μm [49].

As such, the surgical resection is advised for pedunculated MP with Haggitt level 4 and for sessile MP with Sm3 lesion and SMI of more than 1000 μm.

The study done by Toh *et al.* showed that a width of invasion more than 11.5 mm and an area of SMI more than 35 mm^2 were significant predictors for LNM [50]; however, this study was limited by its small sample size and retrospective nature.

4.2 Margin of resection

The positive margin of resection has been defined differently in various literature as tumor <1 mm or < 2 mm or within the cautery of the resection margin [2, 14, 51]. The study has shown that there is increased adverse oncological outcomes if tumor cell is at or near the resection margin [52–55]. In a study done by Hassan *et al.*, it was shown that the patient with positive resection margin had a higher residual and recurrent disease rate and higher rate of hematogenous metastasis and cancer-related mortality [52]. The another study done by Cooper *et al.* showed that there was an increased rate of recurrence of up to 33% when the resection margin was ≤1 mm [54]. Based on the recent scientific evidence, we suggest that 1 mm cutoff margin be a suitable positive margin.

4.3 Tumor differentiation

The tumor differentiation has been categorized into three grades based on the degree of glandular differentiation: grade 1 (well-differentiated), grade 2 (moderately differentiated), and grade 3 (poorly differentiated). The neoplastic lesions with poor differentiation have been shown to be associated with a significantly higher incidence of lymphatic spread and cancer-related mortality [56].

4.4 Lymphovascular invasion

Lymphovascular invasion (LVI) is another important poor prognostic indicator and predictor of patient outcome. The presence of LVI in MP has been associated with an increased risk of regional LNM [56].

4.5 Tumor budding

A single or cluster of up to 5 tumor cells at the advancing front of the tumor has been defined as tumor budding [51, 57]. This has been regarded as a significant risk factor for LNM [56].

4.6 Histological tumor type

A higher risk of LNM has also been found in the MP with cribriform or micro-papillary variants [58, 59]. Moreover, the neoplastic lesions with mucinous or signet ring cells are also associated with a poor prognosis, requiring the surgical resection [60, 61].

The representative endoscopic pictures of the colorectal polyps with regard to the SMI are shown in the **Figures 4–8**.

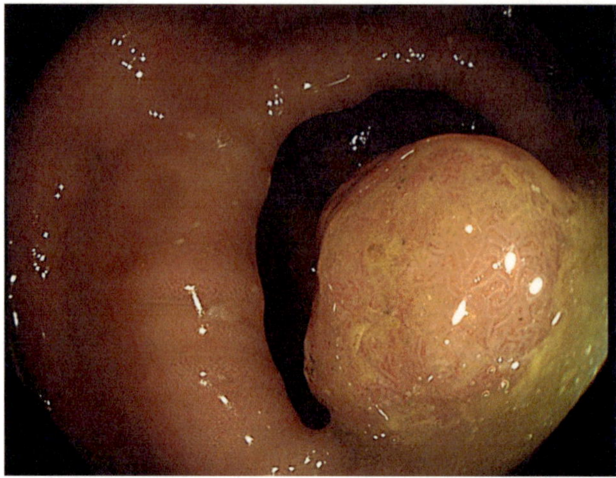

Figure 4.
Large sessile adenomatous polyp; histopathology report showed no SMI.

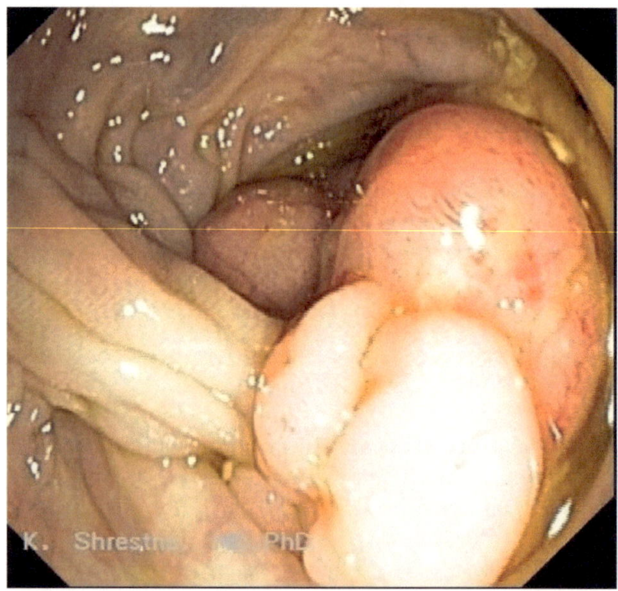

Figure 5.
Pedunculated adenomatous polyp; histopathology report showed no SMI.

5. Management of malignant colorectal polyp (MP)

The management of patients with MP requires a multidisciplinary team approach with the involvement of endoscopists, surgeons, gastrointestinal pathologists, radiologists, and medical oncologists. The flowchart of the proposed algorithm of MP is shown in the **Figure 9**.

Once a colonoscopy reveals a colorectal polyp suggestive of MP, the first critical decision would be to decide whether to resect the polyp completely endoscopically.

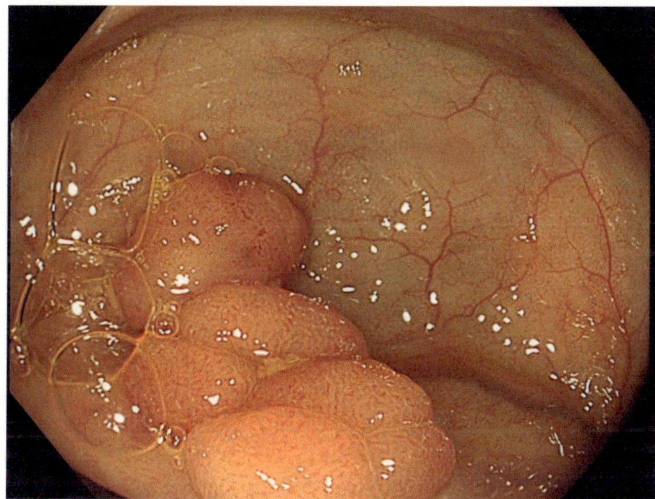

Figure 6.
Sessile polyp with borad base with lobular surface; histopathology report showed MP with superficial SMI.

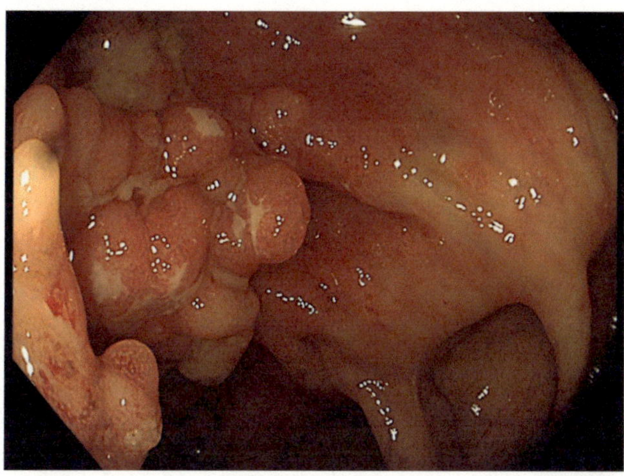

Figure 7.
Laterally spread tumor—granular (LST-G); histopathology report showed MP with deep SMI.

Depending on the nature of the polyp and availability of expertise, the endoscopic removal of MP can be done by conventional snare polypectomy, endoscopic mucosal resection (EMR), endoscopic submucosal dissection (ESD), or other advanced polypectomy technique, such as endoscopic full-thickness resection [16].

The polyps thought to be benign on endoscopy during endoscopic resection have been found to be MP after histopathological evaluation in many instances, and the management of such MP detected after endoscopic resection is difficult because it involves the risk of residual or recurrent disease and of LNM and the patients' surgical risk [12, 22, 62]. Depending upon the morphological, endoscopic, and histological prognostic features, MP is stratified into high- and low-risk polyps. The high-risk features of the MP include poor differentiation, presence of LVI, deep SMI, positive

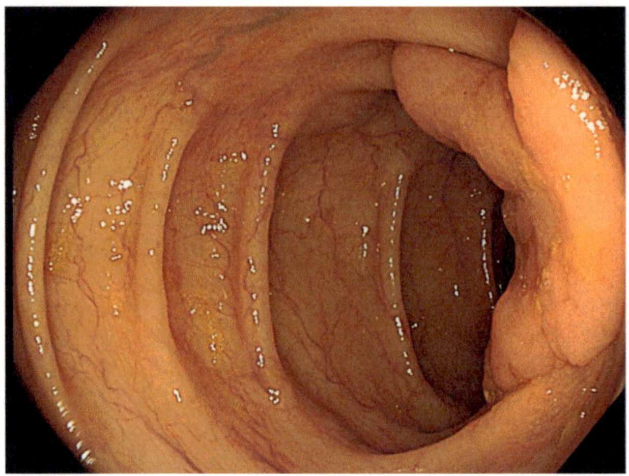

Figure 8.
Laterally spread tumor—non-granular (LST-NG); histopathology report showed MP with deep SMI.

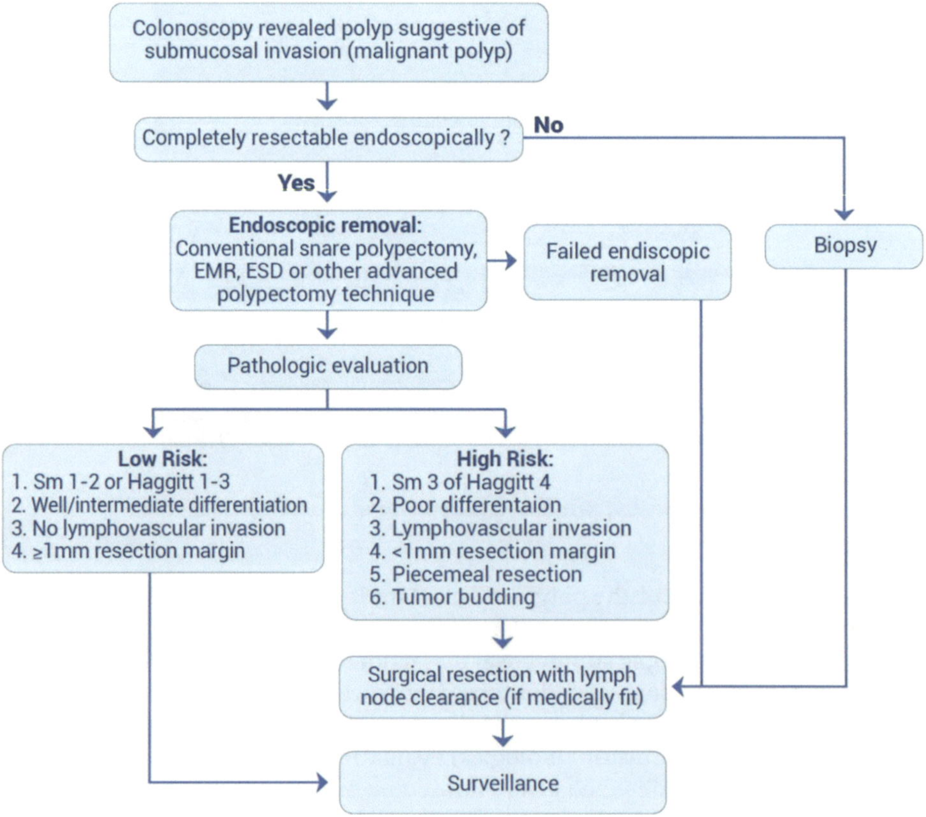

Figure 9.
Proposed algorithm for the management of MP.

margin, piecemeal resection, or tumor budding. Such MPs with high-risk features should undergo surgical resection with lymph node clearance, if medically fit [12, 13, 22, 62]. In the case of the MPs with low-risk features, the endoscopic resection is considered curative and should undergo a surveillance program with regular colonoscopies to detect early recurrence and minimize the risk of metachronous disease. It has been suggested that the surveillance be performed 3–6 months after endoscopic removal of the MP, with the subsequent evaluations to be done based upon the risk and findings [13, 22, 62, 63].

The polyps with certain morphological features associated with a relative high risk of superficial SMI include the polyps with depressed morphology (Paris IIc), LST-NG with depression or bulky sessile appearance (Paris Is component), and LST-G with dominant nodules [26]. Moreover, the risk also increases with lesions ≥20 mm and LSTs located in the right colon, rectosigmoid, and rectum [13, 26].

En-bloc endoscopic resection is needed while removing the probable superficial SMI, because piecemeal resection results in fragmented tissue specimens that compromise the accurate histological assessment. For pedunculated MPs with features suggestive of superficial SMI (Haggitt level 1–3) [16, 60], conventional snare polypectomy is considered adequate for the en-bloc resection and is regarded as curative when the histopathology report and margins are favorable [60]. In the case of large polyp, the snare should be placed closer to the bowel wall than to the head of polyp, in order to obtain the cancer-free resection margin [64].

For the non-pedunculated polyp, the polyp size determines the type of the endoscopic method used for the en-bloc resection [13]. For the lesions ≤20 mm in size, EMR may achieve en-bloc resection, during which the additional margin of normal tissue is snared around the polyp. On the other hand, for the lesions >20 mm in size, ESD is required to achieve en-bloc resection. ESD is associated with a higher en-bloc and curative resection rate and lower risk of recurrence [65], whereas EMR is associated with a higher risk of potential complications and failure during the en-bloc resection of polyps >20 mm [66]. However, ESD is a technically more complex procedure and is associated with a steep learning curve with higher rate of serious adverse events [62, 67].

The polyps with NICE type 3, Kudo class V, surface ulceration without prior manipulation (i.e. biopsies or resection attempts), or stiffness of the lesion and colon wall are suggestive of deep SMI and are associated with LNM and need for surgery [68, 69]. For pedunculated MP, it was found that Haggitt level 4 invasion, LVI, muscularis mucosae type B (incompletely or completely disrupted), poorly differentiated clusters, and tumor budding were the high-risk histologic features, which need the surgery [70]. In another study, it was shown that even in high-risk MP, a high proportion of patients do not have evidence of residual disease in the bowel wall or in the draining lymph nodes [56]. It seems prudent to recommend surgical resection only if 2 or more high risk histological features are present (risk of nodal metastasis: 23.3%); in cases where only one risk feature is present, the estimated risk of nodal metastasis is 4.5% [71].

Certain polyps have indeterminate characteristics that include the following: lesions with endoscopic appearance suggestive of deep SMI yet negative for invasive cancer on biopsies [72, 73], lesions with equivocal endoscopic appearance for deep SMI, and lesions with equivocal biopsy results (i.e., histopathology showing "at least" high-grade dysplasia yet deeper invasion cannot be excluded based on the limited sample). These polyps need to be properly evaluated and managed in a high-volume center with expertise in both endoscopic imaging and resection of complex polyps.

6. Surveillance

There should be a proper colonoscopic surveillance strategy for MPs with both postsurgical resection as well as endoscopic resection [14]. The patients of MP with high-risk features but without the involvement of lymph node, who underwent the formal oncological resection of colon with lymph node clearance, are regarded as a T1 CRC, and surveillance with colonoscopy should be done at 1 year and repeated in 3 years and then every 5 years if there are no advanced adenomas [14]. If the colonoscopy done at 1 year reveals advanced adenoma, the colonoscopic surveillance should be repeated in 1 year. The cross-sectional imaging, endoscopic surveillance, and serial carcinoembryonic antigen testing should be done as per the National Clinical Practice Guidelines in Oncology, if there is a lymph nodal involvement [14]. For the patients of MP with low-risk features, who underwent the endoscopic resection, the surveillance colonoscopy should be done at 3 months, then at 1, 3, and 5 years, as recommended by the US Multi-Society Task Force on Colorectal Cancer and the American Cancer Society [74].

7. Conclusion

With the increasing use of colonoscopy, many patients having MPs are being diagnosed. The management of MP is challenging and begins with the accurate endoscopic assessment of the polyp. The IEE helps to differentiate the superficial and deep SMI of the neoplastic lesion and identify the MP amenable for endoscopic resection or require formal oncological surgery. The endoscopic resection techniques, such as conventional polypectomy, EMR, or ESD, best suited for each type of polyp, need to be determined. After the endoscopic resection of the polyp, the thorough assessment of histological features is important to determine the possibility of residual tumor, the risk of recurrence, and the risk of lymph node involvement. The presence of high risk features (deep SMI, poor differentiation, LVI, <1 mm resection margin, piecemeal resection, tumor budding) indicates a need for surgical resection with lymph node clearance (if medically fit) in the majority of cases. In case of the MPs with low-risk features, the endoscopic resection is considered adequate and further surveillance is advised; when compared to surgery, endoscopic resection is less costly and associated with improved clinical outcomes and patient satisfaction. Moreover, the final decision about the endoscopic resection versus surgical resection of MP needs to be individualized and should be based not only on polyp related characteristics but also on comorbidities, local resources, expertise availability, and patient's preference. The management of patients with MP requires a multidisciplinary team approach with the involvement of referring physicians, endoscopists, surgeons, pathologists, radiologists, and medical oncologists.

Conflict of interest

The author declares no conflict of interest.

Abbreviations

MP	malignant colorectal polyp
CRC	colorectal cancer
LNM	lymph node metastasis
CIN	chromosomal instability
MSI	microsatellite instability
CIMP	CpG island methylator phenotype
K-ras	Kirsten-ras
APC	adenomatous polyposis coli gene
DCC	deleted on colorectal cancer gene
LOH	loss of heterozygosity
HNPCC	hereditary nonpolyposis colorectal cancer
SMI	submucosal invasion
LST	lateral spreading tumor
LST-G	lateral spreading tumor-granular
LST-NG	lateral spreading tumor-non-granular
IEE	image-enhanced endoscopy
NBI	narrow-band imaging
NICE	narrow-band imaging International Colorectal Endoscopic
JNET	Japan NBI Expert Team
AI	artificial intelligence
EMR	endoscopic mucosal resection
ESD	endoscopic submucosal dissection

Author details

Umid Kumar Shrestha
Department of Gastroenterology, Nepal Mediciti Hospital, Bhaisepati, Lalitpur, Nepal

*Address all correspondence to: umidshrestha@gmail.com

References

[1] Dekker E, Tanis PJ, Vleugels JLA, Kasi PM, Wallace MB. Colorectal cancer. Lancet. 2019;**394**:1467-1480

[2] Mathews AA, Draganov PV, Yang D. Endoscopic management of colorectal polyps: From benign to malignant polyps. World Journal of Gastroenterology. 2021;**13**(9):356-370

[3] Amin MB, Edge S, Greene F, Byrd DR, Brookland RK, Washington MK, et al. AJCC Cancer Staging Manual. 8th ed. New York, NY: Springer; 2017. pp. 252-254

[4] Hackelsberger A, Frühmorgen P, Weiler H, Heller T, Seeliger H, Junghanns K. Endoscopic polypectomy and management of colorectal adenomas with invasive carcinoma. Endoscopy. 1995;**27**:153-158

[5] Netzer P, Forster C, Biral R, Ruchti C, Neuweiler J, Stauffer E, et al. Risk factor assessment of endoscopically removed malignant colorectal polyp. Gut. 1998;**43**:669-674

[6] Coverlizza S, Risio M, Ferrari A, Fenoglio-Preiser CM, Rossini FP. Colorectal adenomas containing invasive carcinoma. Pathologic assessment of lymph node metastatic potential. Cancer. 1989;**64**:1937-1947

[7] Tateishi Y, Nakanishi Y, Taniguchi H, Shimoda T, Umemura S. Pathological prognostic factors predicting lymph node metastasis in submucosal invasive (T1) colorectal carcinoma. Modern Pathology. 2010;**23**:1068-1072

[8] Klimeck L, Heisser T, Hoffmeister M. Hermann Brenner colorectal cancer: A health and economic problem. Best Practice & Research Clinical Gastroenterology. 2023;**2023**:101839

[9] Kuipers EJ, Rösch T, Bretthauer M. Colorectal cancer screening–optimizing current strategies and new directions. Nature Reviews. Clinical Oncology. 2013;**10**:130-142

[10] Armaghany T, Wilson JD, Chu Q, Mills G. Genetic alterations in colorectal cancer. Gastrointestinal Cancer Research. 2012;**5**(1):19-27

[11] Elisa De Palma FD, Pol J, Kroemer G, Maria Chiara Maiuri MC, Salvatore F. The molecular hallmarks of the serrated pathway in colorectal cancer. Cancer (Basel). 2019;**11**(7):1017

[12] Labianca R, Nordlinger B, Beretta GD, Mosconi S, Mandalà M, Cervantes A, et al., editors. Early colon cancer:ESMO Clinical Practice Guidelines for diagnosis, treatment and follow-up. Annals of Oncology. 2013;**24**:vi64-vi72

[13] Shaukat A, Kaltenbach T, Dominitz JA, Robertson DJ, Anderson JC, Cruise M, et al. Endoscopic recognition and management strategies for malignant colorectal polyps: Recommendations of the US multi-society task force on colorectal cancer. Gastroenterology. 2020;**159**:1916-1934

[14] Teo NZ, Wijaya R, Ngu JC. Management of malignant colonic polyps. Journal of Gastrointestinal Oncology. 2020;**11**:469-474

[15] Backes Y, Schwartz MP, Ter Borg F, Wolfhagen FHJ, Groen JN, et al. Multicentre prospective evaluation of real-time optical diagnosis of T1 colorectal cancer in large

non-pedunculated colorectal polyps using narrow band imaging (the OPTICAL study). Gut. 2019;**68**:271-279

[16] Rex DK, Shaukat A, Wallace MB. Optimal management of malignant polyps, from endoscopic assessment and resection to decisions about surgery. Clinical Gastroenterology and Hepatology. 2019;**17**:1428-1437

[17] Waye JD, O'Brien MJ. Cancer in polyps. In: Cohen A, Winawer S, editors. Cancer of the Colon, Rectum and Anus. New York: McGraw-Hill; 1994. pp. 465-476

[18] O'Brien MJ, Winawer SJ, Waye JD. Colorectal polyps. In: Winawer S, editor. Management of Gastrointestinal Diseases. New York: Gower Inc.; 1992

[19] Cranley JP, Petras RE, Carey WD, et al. When is endoscopic polypectomy adequate therapy for colonic polyps containing invasive carcinoma? Gastroenterology. 1987;**91**:419-427

[20] Rossini FP, Ferrari A, Coverlizza S, et al. Large bowel adenomas containing carcinoma: A diagnostic and therapeutic approach. International Journal of Colorectal Disease. 1988;**3**:47-52

[21] Sugihara K, Muto T, Morioka Y. Management of patients with invasive carcinoma removed by colonoscopic polypectomy. Diseases of the Colon and Rectum. 1989;**32**:829-834

[22] Williams CB, Whiteway JE, Jass JR. Practical aspects of endoscopic management of malignant polyps. Endoscopy. 1987;**19**:31-37

[23] Christie JP. Polypectomy or colectomy? Management of 106 consecutively encountered colorectal polyps. The American Surgeon. 1988;**54**:93-99

[24] Rembacken BJ, Fujii T, Cairns A, Dixon MF, Yoshida S, Chalmers DM, et al. Flat and depressed colonic neoplasms: A prospective study of 1000 colonoscopies in the UK. Lancet. 2000;**355**:1211-1214

[25] Soetikno RM, Kaltenbach T, Rouse RV, Park W, Maheshwari A, Sato T, et al. Prevalence of nonpolypoid (flat and depressed) colorectal neoplasms in asymptomatic and symptomatic adults. Journal of the American Medical Association. 2008;**299**:1027-1035

[26] Moss A, Bourke MJ, Williams SJ, Hourigan LF, Brown G, Tam W, et al. Endoscopic mucosal resection outcomes and prediction of submucosal cancer from advanced colonic mucosal neoplasia. Gastroenterology. 2011;**140**:1909-1918

[27] Conteduca V, Sansonno D, Russi S, Dammacco F. Precancerous colorectal lesions (Review). International Journal of Oncology. 2013;**43**:973-984

[28] Lopez A, Bouvier AM, Jooste V, Cottet V, Romain G, Faivre J, et al. Outcomes following polypectomy for malignant colorectal polyps are similar to those following surgery in the general population. Gut. 2019;**68**:111-117

[29] Bogie RMM, Veldman MHJ, Snijders LARS, Winkens B, Kaltenbach T, Masclee AAM, et al. Endoscopic subtypes of colorectal laterally spreading tumors (LSTs) and the risk of submucosal invasion: A meta-analysis. Endoscopy. 2018;**50**:263-282

[30] Burgess NG, Hourigan LF, Zanati SA, Brown GJ, Singh R, Williams SJ, et al. Risk stratification for covert invasive cancer among patients referred for colonic endoscopic mucosal resection: A Large Multicenter Cohort. Gastroenterology. 2017;**153**:732-742

[31] Bettington M, Walker N, Clouston A, Brown I, Leggett B, Whitehall V. The serrated pathway to colorectal carcinoma:Current concepts and challenges. Histopathology. 2013;**62**:367-386

[32] Puig I, López-Cerón M, Arnau A, et al. Accuracy of the narrow-band imaging international colorectal endoscopic classification system in identification of deep invasion in colorectal polyps. Gastroenterology. 2019;**156**:75-87

[33] Shahidi N, Vosko S, van Hattem WA, Sidhu M, Bourke MJ. Optical evaluation:The crux for effective management of colorectal neoplasia. Therapeutic Advances in Gastroenterology. 2020;**13**:1756

[34] Sano Y, Kobayashi M, Kozu T, et al. Development and clinical application of a narrow band imaging (NBI) system with built-in narrow-band RGB filters. Stomach Intestine. 2001;**36**:1283-1287

[35] Sano Y. NBI story. Early Colorectal Cancer. 2007;**11**:91-92

[36] Yasushi Sano Y, Shinji Tanaka S, Shin-ei Kudo S, Shoichi Saito S, Takahisa Matsuda T, Yoshiki Wada Y, et al. Narrow-band imaging (NBI) magnifying endoscopic classification of colorectal tumors proposed by the Japan. NBI Expert Team. 2016;**28**(5):526-533

[37] Hewett DG, Kaltenbach T, Sano Y, et al. Validation of a simple classification system for endoscopic diagnosis of small colorectal polyps using narrow-band imaging. Gastroenterology. 2012;**143**:599-607

[38] Iwatate M, Sano Y, Tanaka S, Kudo SE, Saito S, Matsuda T, et al. Japan NBI expert team (JNET) validation study for development of the Japan NBI expert team classification of colorectal lesions. Digestive Endoscopy. 2018;**30**:642-651

[39] Kudo S, Hirota S, Nakajima T, Hosobe S, Kusaka H, Kobayashi T, et al. Colorectal tumours and pit pattern. Journal of Clinical Pathology. 1994;**47**:880-885

[40] Ali SM, Uma S, Liu J, Li YQ, Zuo XL. Kudo's pit pattern classification for colorectal neoplasms: A meta-analysis. World Journal of Gastroenterology. 2014;**20**(35):12649-12656

[41] Togashi K, Konishi F, Ishizuka T, Sato T, Senba S, Kanazawa K. Efficacy of magnifying endoscopy in the differential diagnosis of neoplastic and non-neoplastic polyps of the large bowel. Diseases of the Colon and Rectum. 1999;**42**:1602-1608

[42] Lui TKL, Wong KKY, Mak LLY, Ko MKL, Tsao SKK, Leung WK. Endoscopic prediction of deeply submucosal invasive carcinoma with use of artificial intelligence. Endoscopic International Open. 2019;**7**:E514-E520

[43] Luo X, Wang J, Han Z, et al. Artificial intelligence-enhanced white-light colonoscopy with attention guidance predicts colorectal cancer invasion depth. Gastrointestinal Endoscopy. 2021;**94**:627-638

[44] Kudo SE, Ichimasa K, Villard B, et al. Artificial intelligence system to determine risk of T1 colorectal cancer metastasis to lymph node. Gastroenterology. 2021;**160**:1075-1084

[45] Haggitt RC, Glotzbach RE, Soffer EE, Wruble LD. Prognostic factors in colorectal carcinomas arising in adenomas: Implications for lesions removed by endoscopic polypectomy. Gastroenterology. 1985;**89**:328-336

[46] Kikuchi R, Takano M, Takagi K, Fujimoto N, Nozaki R, Fujiyoshi T, et al.

Management of early invasive colorectal cancer. Risk of recurrence and clinical guidelines. Diseases of the Colon and Rectum. 1995;**38**:1286-1295

[47] Kitajima K, Fujimori T, Fujii S, Takeda J, Ohkura Y, Kawamata H, et al. Correlations between lymph node metastasis and depth of submucosal invasion in submucosal invasive colorectal carcinoma: A Japanese collaborative study. Journal of Gastroenterology. 2004;**39**:534-543

[48] Nivatvongs S, Rojanasakul A, Reiman HM, Dozois RR, Wolff BG, Pemberton JH, et al. The risk of lymph node metastasis in colorectal polyps with invasive adenocarcinoma. Diseases of the Colon and Rectum. 1991;**34**:323-328

[49] Beaton C, Twine CP, Williams GL, Radcliffe AG. Systematic review and meta-analysis of histopathological factors influencing the risk of lymph node metastasis in early colorectal cancer. Colorectal Disease. 2013;**15**:788-797

[50] Toh EW, Brown P, Morris E, Botterill I, Quirke P. Area of submucosal invasion and width of invasion predicts lymph node metastasis in pT1 colorectal cancers. Diseases of the Colon and Rectum. 2015;**58**:393-400

[51] Berg KB, Telford JJ, Gentile L, Schaeffer DF. Re-examining the 1-mm margin and submucosal depth of invasion:A review of 216 malignant colorectal polyps. Virchows Archiv. 2020;**476**:863-870

[52] Hassan C, Zullo A, Risio M, Rossini FP, Morini S. Histologic risk factors and clinical outcome in colorectal malignant polyp: A pooled-data analysis. Diseases of the Colon and Rectum. 2005;**48**:1588-1596

[53] Ueno H, Mochizuki H, Hashiguchi Y, Shimazaki H, Aida S, Hase K, et al. Risk factors for an adverse outcome in early invasive colorectal carcinoma. Gastroenterology. 2004;**127**:385-394

[54] Cooper HS, Deppisch LM, Gourley WK, Kahn EI, Lev R, Manley PN, et al. Endoscopically removed malignant colorectal polyps:Clinicopathologic correlations. Gastroenterology. 1995;**108**:1657-1665

[55] Boenicke L, Fein M, Sailer M, Isbert C, Germer CT, Thalheimer A. The concurrence of histologically positive resection margins and sessile morphology is an important risk factor for lymph node metastasis after complete endoscopic removal of malignant colorectal polyps. International Journal of Colorectal Disease. 2010;**25**:433-438

[56] Brown IS, Bettington ML, Bettington A, Miller G, Rosty C. Adverse histological features in malignant colorectal polyps: A contemporary series of 239 cases. Journal of Clinical Pathology. 2016;**69**:292-299

[57] Kuo E, Wang K, Liu X. A focused review on advances in risk stratification of malignant polyps. Gastroenterology Research. 2020;**13**:163-183

[58] Egashira Y, Yoshida T, Hirata I, Hamamoto N, Akutagawa H, Takeshita A, et al. Analysis of pathological risk factors for lymph node metastasis of submucosal invasive colon cancer. Modern Pathology. 2004;**17**:503-511

[59] Xu F, Xu J, Lou Z, Di M, Wang F, Hu H, et al. Micropapillary component in colorectal carcinoma is associated with lymph node metastasis in T1 and T2 stages and decreased survival time in TNM stages I and II. The American Journal of Surgical Pathology. 2009;**33**:1287-1292

[60] Williams JG, Pullan RD, Hill J, Horgan PG, Salmo E, Buchanan GN, et al. Association of Coloproctology of Great Britain and Ireland. Management of the malignant colorectal polyp: ACPGBI position statement. Colorectal Disease. 2013;**15**:1-38

[61] Watanabe T, Muro K, Ajioka Y, Hashiguchi Y, Ito Y, Saito Y, et al. Japanese Society for Cancer of the Colon and Rectum (JSCCR) guidelines 2016 for the treatment of colorectal cancer. International Journal of Clinical Oncology. 2018;**23**:1-34

[62] Aarons CB, Shanmugan S, Bleier JI. Management of malignant colon polyps:Current status and controversies. World Journal of Gastroenterology. 2014;**20**:16178-16183

[63] Bartel MJ, Brahmbhatt BS, Wallace MB. Management of colorectal T1 carcinoma treated by endoscopic resection from the Western perspective. Digestive Endoscopy. 2016;**28**:330-341

[64] Ciocalteu A, Gheonea DI, Saftoiu A, Streba L, Dragoescu NA, Tenea-Cojan TS. Current strategies for malignant pedunculated colorectal polyps. World Journal of Gastrointestinal Oncology. 2018;**10**:465-475

[65] Fujiya M, Tanaka K, Dokoshi T, Tominaga M, Ueno N, Inaba Y, et al. Efficacy and adverse events of EMR and endoscopic submucosal dissection for the treatment of colon neoplasms: A meta-analysis of studies comparing EMR and endoscopic submucosal dissection. Gastrointestinal Endoscopy. 2015;**81**:583-595

[66] Chandan S, Khan SR, Kumar A, Mohan BP, Ramai D, Kassab LL, et al. Efficacy and histologic accuracy of underwater versus conventional endoscopic mucosal resection for large (>20 mm) colorectal polyps: A comparative review and meta-analysis. Gastrointestinal Endoscopy. 2021;**97**(3):471-482

[67] Yang D, Othman M, Draganov PV. Endoscopic mucosal resection vs endoscopic submucosal dissection for Barrett's Esophagus and colorectal neoplasia. Clinical Gastroenterology and Hepatology. 2019;**17**:1019-1028

[68] Hayashi N, Tanaka S, Hewett DG, Kaltenbach TR, Sano Y, Ponchon T, et al. Endoscopic prediction of deep submucosal invasive carcinoma: Validation of the narrow-band imaging international colorectal endoscopic (NICE) classification. Gastrointestinal Endoscopy. 2013;**78**:625-632

[69] Rastogi A, Keighley J, Singh V, Callahan P, Bansal A, Wani S, et al. High accuracy of narrow band imaging without magnification for the real-time characterization of polyp histology and its comparison with high-definition white light colonoscopy: A prospective study. The American Journal of Gastroenterology. 2009;**104**:2422-2430

[70] Backes Y, Elias SG, Groen JN, Schwartz MP, et al. Dutch T1 CRC working group. Histologic factors associated with need for surgery in patients with pedunculated T1 colorectal carcinomas. Gastroenterology. 2018;**154**:1647-1659

[71] Saraivaa S, Rosaa I, Fonsecab R, Pereira AD. Colorectal malignant polyps: A modern approach. Annals of Gastroenterology. 2022;**35**(1):17-27

[72] Vosko S, Bourke MJ. Gross morphology predicts the presence and pattern of invasive cancer in laterally spreading tumors: Don't overlook the overview! Gastrointestinal Endoscopy. 2020;**92**:1095-1097

[73] Ferlitsch M, Moss A, Hassan C, Bhandari P, Dumonceau JM, Paspatis G, et al. Colorectal polypectomy and endoscopic mucosal resection (EMR): European Society of Gastrointestinal Endoscopy (ESGE) clinical guideline. Endoscopy. 2017;**49**:270-297

[74] Winawer SJ, Zauber AG, Fletcher RH, Stillman JS, O'Brien MJ, Levin B, et al. Guidelines for colonoscopy surveillance after polypectomy: A consensus update by the US multi-society task force on colorectal Cancer and the American Cancer Society. Gastroenterology. 2006;**130**:1872-1885

Chapter 6

The Evolving Landscape of Colonoscopy: Recent Developments and Complication Management

Riya Patel, Shivani Patel, Ilyas Momin and Shreeraj Shah

Abstract

Colorectal cancer is globally recognized as the third most prevalent cancer, highlighting the crucial role of colonoscopy in diagnosis and therapeutic interventions. This medical procedure has demonstrated its effectiveness in preventing colorectal cancer and investigating a wide range of gastrointestinal symptoms. It has long been acknowledged as the gold standard for screening colorectal cancer. The primary objective of this analysis is to outline diverse range of complications associated with preparatory phase of colonoscopy, especially among hospitalized patients, including those with potentially life-threatening conditions. The ultimate aim is to elucidate strategies to prevent complications during the preparatory phase of colonoscopy. The real-time visual feed produced by endoscopic camera allows for the detection of abnormal growth of the colonic wall. This capability facilitates the assessment, biopsy, and removal of mucosal lesions through various biopsy instruments accessible via specialized channels. With its multifaceted utility, colonoscopy has become a frontline approach in making colorectal cancer a preventable and early-detectable disease over the past few decades. Common complications associated with colonoscopy include occurrences like vomiting, nosebleeds, abdominal pain, and acute diarrhoea. This review primarily focuses on developments that have transpired over the past five years, leading to changes in multiple aspects of colonoscopy.

Keywords: gastroenterology, diagnostics, colonoscopy, colon diseases, colonoscope, complication

1. Introduction

In today's contemporary medicine, a colonoscopy is an essential procedure. This approach is essential for saving lives in both immediate and future situations because of its adaptability and usefulness. It is applicable to both cancerous and noncancerous disorders, such as colon impactions, sigmoid volvulus infections, and gastrointestinal hemorrhage. Performing a colonoscopy for screening purposes is crucial in identifying and addressing colorectal cancers in their early stages. This procedure plays a significant role in guiding the course of cancer treatment, assisting in the planning of surgical measures [1]. Recent colonoscopies face a number of difficulties because of the unique characteristics of the colon, including the possibility of a highly repetitive sigmoid colon in certain people. In certain cases, the transverse colon forms an M shape and goes down into the pelvis. The colon's mostly round shape leads to a semi-circular pattern within the scope after a few twists and further advancement increases the risk of forming a larger loop. At the same time, the tip of the scope does not proceed forward [2].

2. Basics of colonoscopy

The United States performs over 15 million colonoscopies annually, and it is estimated that these procedures lower the overall risk of dying from colorectal cancer by more than 60% [3]. Because of advancements in upper endoscopy, colonoscopy was initially introduced in the 1960s [4]. Colonoscopy is a diagnosis and curative technique used to assess the distal part of the small intestine and the large intestine. The procedure is carried out with the use of a versatile, hand-held tube-like instrument known as a colonoscope. It includes an attached high-definition camera at its tip and auxiliary channels that enable the insertion of tools and liquids to clean the colonoscope lens and the mucosa of the colon [5]. The imagery captured by the camera and displayed on the screen aids in identifying irregularities and excessive growth on the colon wall. Consequently, this technology enables the assessment, sampling, and elimination of mucosal lesions using various biopsy tools accessible through additional channels. To detect and treat colorectal cancer, a colonoscopy is essential. It is a suggested screening method for people with risk factors, such as a family history of cancer or tumors, and is the best way to find cancerous colonies [6]. Progressive advancements in imaging technology, the evolution of guidelines, heightened awareness, and expanded access have collectively contributed to increased utilization and broader utility. In this review, we will explore the various kinds, uses, and potential complications of colonoscopies, along with their management strategies, future advancements, and the scope of their application. The colon and colonoscopy are shown in **Figure 1**.

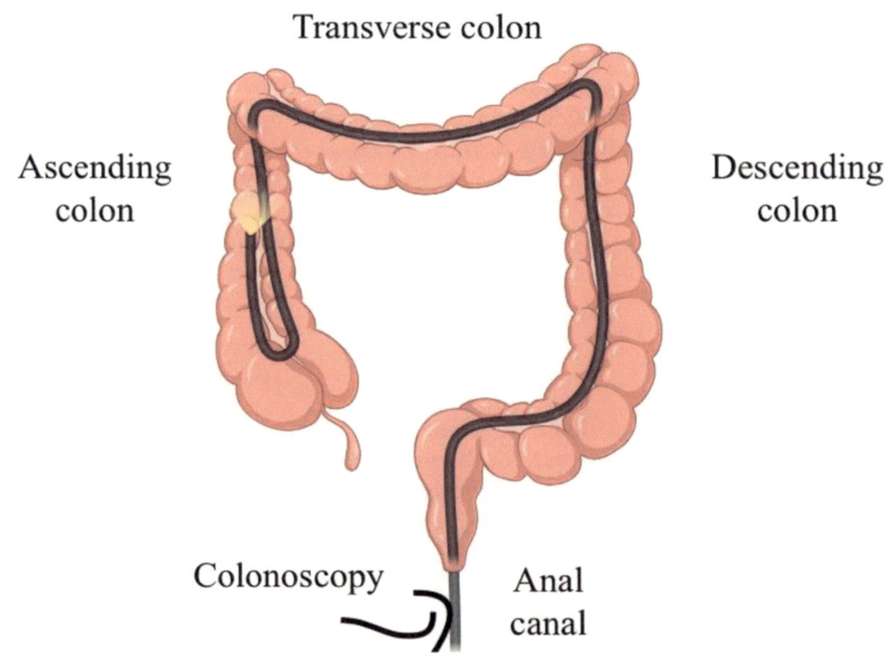

Figure 1.
Colon and colonoscopy.

2.1 History and the need for colonoscopy

Colon cancer is more likely to strike an older person. Although it can be identified in younger persons, it is far more frequent after the age of 45 years. The cause of the rising incidence of colon cancer in people aged under 45 years is unknown [7]. A background of adenomatous polyps elevates the likelihood of developing colon cancer, particularly in cases involving large polyps, multiple polyps, or those displaying dysplasia. Following the identification of polyps and the assessment of results, the gastroenterologist will suggest a screening timetable tailored to individual-specific risk factors [8].

2.1.1 Family past with cancer or polyps in the colon

Although the majority of colon cancers occur in individuals without a family history, up to one-third of individuals diagnosed with colon cancer have relatives who have also experienced the disease. Adenomatous polyps, the type of polyps that have the potential to turn cancerous, have been linked to a greater chance of developing colon cancer in family members. The reason for this is not fully apparent. Because of heredity, the environment, or a mix of both, cancer may be passed down in families.

2.1.2 Personal history of inflammatory bowel disease (IBD)

Suffering from IBD such as ulcerative colitis or Crohn's disease heightens the likelihood of developing colon cancer. It is essential to note that IBD should not be confused with irritable bowel syndrome (IBS), which does not seem to elevate the risk of colon cancer. Individuals with IBD might necessitate earlier initiation of colon cancer screening and more frequent screenings [9].

2.1.3 Signs of colon cancer

Although most early cases of colon cancer are asymptomatic, anybody experiencing symptoms such as bleeding in the feces, bleeding from the rectal area, pain in the stomach, and unexpected weight loss should see a gastroenterologist.

2.2 Types of colonoscopies

There are two kinds of colonoscopies: screening and diagnostic.

2.2.1 Screening colonoscopy

A screening colonoscopy is a proactive examination performed to ensure the colon's good health. If a person has a first-degree relative with a medical history of colon polyps or cancer, has potential indicators for colorectal cancer, or has had a colon polyp or cancer in the past, they may need a preventative colonoscopy for screening purposes.

2.2.2 Diagnostic colonoscopy

Diagnostic colonoscopy may be required if there is a significant family record of colon tumors or possible symptoms. It might require a diagnostic colonoscopy if a person experiences symptoms such as bleeding from the rectum or in the feces, persistent abdominal pain, persistent alteration in bowel movements for an extended period, iron-deficiency anemia, and a history of polyps in the colon or cancer in family members.

2.3 Method

The effectiveness of various colonoscopy surveillance approaches relies on specific parameters that determine their viability in comparison to white light colonoscopy. Two important performance metrics are the colonoscopy withdrawal time, which shows how long it takes to remove the colonoscope, and the local intubation rate, which shows what proportion of the colon can be viewed [10]. There are five popular types of colonoscopy methods.

2.3.1 Virtual colonoscopy (VC)

This quickly evolving method uses data from computed tomography (CT) scans to produce 2D and 3D pictures of both the rectum and the colon. This technique is occasionally known as computed tomographic colonography [11]. Rather than employing the traditional approach, VC creates a picture of the rectum or colon using x-rays, and conventional colonoscopies are used to examine it. This method is favored due to its noninvasive nature, eliminating patient discomfort and obviating the need for sedation. Unlike standard colonoscopies that involve sedatives and may require a recovery period before normal activities can be resumed, virtual colonoscopy offers a more convenient alternative [12]. VC was introduced as a colorectal cancer screening procedure in the United States by the American Cancer Society, the American College of Radiology, and the U.S. Multi-Society Task Force for Colorectal Cancer. For the last decade, hospitals have extensively utilized this approach. Research conducted by Agha et al. revealed that virtual colonoscopy exhibited a sensitivity and specificity of 97 and 100%, respectively, in identifying polyps larger than 1 cm. Consequently, this approach has the capability to detect a greater number of lesions compared to conventional colonoscopy. The necessity for invasive procedures would decrease with the introduction of VC. Despite being less costly, this method can still result in false-positive outcomes, lowering sensitivity to 93%. A false positive will lead to more needless steps and processes [13].

2.3.2 Chromo-colonoscopy using dye-based techniques

In this method, a colon is sprayed with a dye solution. Applying this dye increases the likelihood of identifying nonpolypoid lesions, which increases the detection rate of adenomas [14]. Apart from the dye spray, this method uses a standard colonoscopy instrument. Various dyes are employed based on preference and intended objectives. These dyes fall into three main categories: contrast, absorptive, or reactive. Contrast dyes, such as indigo carmine, permeate irregularities and accumulate on polyps, enhancing visibility during the procedure [15]. Crystal violet is one example of an absorbent dye that penetrates epithelial cells and makes it easier to differentiate between tumors and infections. Absorptive dye requires initial treatment, such as mucus clearance from the mucosa wall, compared to contrast dye [16]. Responsive staining, such as Congo red, employs chemical reactions to draw attention to certain features inside the tissue. Indigo carmine is the most often used contrast dye because it is affordable, nonhazardous, and easy to use [17]. Unlike traditional colonoscopy, this kind of colonoscopy, which takes random specimens, permits targeted biopsies.

Compared to traditional colonoscopy, this method greatly increases the possibility of discovery because it can differentiate between lesions and polyps and normal mucosa. Wu et al. conducted a study demonstrating that the application of dye-based chromo-colonoscopy resulted in higher sensitivity (95%) compared to conventional colonoscopy. However, the sensitivity varied based on the type of dye utilized. The use of indigo carmine exhibited superior sensitivity compared to methylene blue (74%), but it also indicated lower specificity. Specifically, indigo carmine had a specificity of 91%, whereas methylene blue had a specificity of 92% [18]. The differences in the colors' ability to help physicians distinguish tumors from their surrounding mucosa, which makes polyp identification simpler, may be the cause of the discrepancy in outcomes. The adoption of this technique has been inconsistent, likely due to a steep learning curve. In clinical use, it has not become a widely accepted alternative for conventional colonoscopy, in part due to the unpleasant and lengthy nature of dye application. Furthermore, some research indicates that some dyes, such as methylene blue, can be cancerous [16].

2.3.3 Electronic chromo-colonoscopy

Narrow band imaging (NBI), flexible spectrum imaging color enhancement (FICE), and i-scan digital contrast (i-scan) are the three primary forms of electronic chromo-colonoscopy. These methods all provide a mucosal contrast with the colon's blood vessels. Among the three approaches discussed, NBI has been extensively studied. When compared to traditional colonoscopy, electronic chromo-colonoscopy typically has a sensitivity of 91%, meaning that polyps or lesions are less likely to be missed [19].

2.3.3.1 Narrow band imaging (NBI)

NBI is dependent on hemoglobin's ability to absorb light, which accentuates the mucosa's vasculature. However, the light source is filtered such that it only emits the green and blue bands of light, which represent the maxima of hemoglobin's light absorption [20]. The absorption peaks of light in this method occur at 415 nm (blue light) and 540 nm (green light). The vascular mucosa has a combination of green and blue coloration that enhances the visibility of structures and patterns. This method allows for focused biopsies and can distinguish between malignant and benign cells, similar to dye-based chromo-colonoscopy. Interestingly, this method defines the boundaries of lesions without the use of dyes, which can be more convenient for individuals who are allergic to dyes in their bodies. In a 2014 study, the use of NBI for adenomas and polyp detection demonstrated a sensitivity of 98%, indicating its efficiency in detecting lesions, polyps, or adenomas. However, the accuracy of this technique, at 75%, is noticeably lower than that of a conventional colonoscopy [21]. Vişovan and his colleagues recently finished research that indicated elevated rates of polyp and adenoma detection. Numerous studies have been done on the use of NBI, and the bulk of the earlier studies have concluded that it is not a practical solution. Nevertheless, Olympus sells this technique that has been used in clinical settings [19, 22].

2.3.3.2 Flexible spectral imaging color enhancement (FICE)

White light colonoscopy is used in this approach; however, the final picture is digitally altered using algorithms based on spectra emission techniques to change the prominence of specific wavelengths. FICE incorporates optical filters and spectra-estimation technology to generate images from white light colonoscopy at various wavelengths [23, 24]. This method makes vascular and surface structures apparent through magnification, making it easier to distinguish between atypical and typical tissue development. Randomly selected single-wavelength images are designated to the colors blue, green, and red [25]. This enables the creation of an improved color image, utilized for structural and vascular enhancements. The technology includes 10 presets that can be customized further, offering a wide range of wavelength combinations. According to Lami and colleagues, FICE has a higher detection rate than white light colonoscopy, which suggests that it may be a more effective procedure for finding adenomas [26]. Osawa and colleagues conducted a study to explore the potential of FICE as a substitute for traditional colonoscopy. The research revealed that FICE demonstrated effectiveness in screening esophageal and gastric lesions characterized by high color contrast, yielding a notable sensitivity of 88% and specificity of 88% [27, 28]. Nevertheless, FICE has not been thoroughly investigated, preventing its clinical implementation, unlike NBI.

2.3.3.3 i-scan digital contrast

Similar to FICE, i-scan is a new technique that makes use of the pictures from white light colonoscopy. Using three distinct algorithm modes, the user may apply filters to a picture to improve tissue contrast through the use of an i-scan software [29–31]. One of the three functions focuses on surface enhancement, aiming to increase the distinction between light and dark areas. This results in improved visualization and a more thorough examination of the structure of the mucosal surface. According to Bowman and colleagues, surface augmentation makes it easier to identify the boundaries between pathological and normal mucosa. The polyp identification efficiency is increased by using this method. Enhancement of contrast is the second mode. By suppressing the wavelengths of red and green, this produces a blue-tint picture that improves the visualization of the mucosal surface's depth [32]. The use of contrast enhancement is helpful not only in revealing abnormalities that might go unnoticed with exclusive reliance on white light colonoscopy but also in visualizing irregularities. The last mode, known as tone enhancement, involves limiting the red wavelength, thereby improving the visualization of subtle irregularities and the vascular structure within the mucosa. According to Cho and his colleagues, tone enhancement proves to be an effective tool for characterizing previously identified lesions [29, 33, 34]. In a clinical research, Hoffman and collaborators evaluated the efficacy of i-scan versus conventional colonoscopy. The findings from their research indicated a higher detection rate of polyps when using i-scan in comparison to conventional colonoscopy alone. While most studies incorporating i-scan also utilize other techniques, the majority of these combined approaches demonstrate enhanced sensitivity. Therefore, it appears that i-scan may enhance sensitivity, but its effectiveness is most notable when used in combination with other techniques [35].

2.3.4 Autofluorescence imaging (AFI)

The tissue of the colon may include fluorophores such as collagen, nicotinamide, flavin, and porphyrins. They release a naturally occurring fluorescent light that is sometimes referred to as autofluorescence (AF) light when stimulated by light (ultraviolet or short visible light). The light utilized for illumination is shorter in wavelength (500–630 nm) than the light generated by the AF, which results in a pseudocolor image on the colonoscopy display. The emitted fluorescence is contingent on the composition of tissues, the variety of fluorophores, their concentrations, metabolic rates, and spatial distribution. The distinctions in colors enable the AFI system to detect existing lesions. With the help of this approach, blue as well as green lights with wavelengths of around 450 and 550 nm, respectively, are produced by a color filter wheel in rotation. The interference filters built within the colonoscope allow the reading of AF light, reflecting green light onto the filter and eliminating blue light. During the colonoscopy operation, tumors show purple and normal mucosa appears green due to the interference filter. The user can distinguish between abnormalities and normal tissue thanks to this differentiation [29]. There has been research comparing AFI versus white light colonoscopy; however, a study from 2013 found no increase in the rate of detection with AFI [36]. Nevertheless, a 3-year-old study revealed that AFI with a transparent hood boosted polyp identification rates [37, 38].

2.3.5 Capsule colonoscopy endoscopy (CCE)

Initially presented in 2007 as a substitute for conventional colonoscopy, this device requires the patient to ingest a capsule to initiate the imaging process. Three collimated x-ray beams from a rotating source scan the colon as the capsule passes through. Rapid recovery is enabled by the photographic storage's reliance on radio frequencies (RF) and wireless data transfer via a microcontroller. Within a few seconds, the system traces the 3D position and orientation of the capsule within the surrounding colon. Notably, the capsule features optical domes on both ends, providing a more comprehensive view of the lumen compared to conventional colonoscopy [39]. From these initial-generation gadgets, the capsule has undergone additional development. Presently produced in the United States by Medtronic, the second generation devices (CCE-2) contain cameras with a 172° wider field of vision, which results in a 354° field of view. In comparison to CCE-1, which has a 154-degree field of view, this one is significantly bigger. Presently, the CCE device has been employed to address incomplete colonoscopies, detect polyps, and examine inflammatory bowel disease. Incomplete colonoscopy may occur when only a portion of the colon is imaged, potentially resulting in missed lesions or polyps. VC is often employed in cases of incomplete colonoscopies to visualize large polyps and masses in the colon. However, an analysis of 14 studies found that CCE-2 is superior to both CCE and VC for polyp visualization [40]. Yung and colleagues conducted a review of multiple studies examining the efficacy of CCE and CCE-2 in detecting polyps. The findings indicated that for polyps smaller than 6 mm, CCE and CCE-2 demonstrated an overall sensitivity of 58 and 86%, respectively. Additionally, they exhibited overall specificities of 85.7 and 88.1% [41]. As a result, CCE-2 is more useful in the identification of polyps, and it excretes capsules at a somewhat higher rate than CCE. CCE is favored over virtual colonoscopy because of its superior detection rates and the potential adverse effects of x-rays on the human body. However, a notable drawback of capsule endoscopy is its time-consuming and labor-intensive nature that could impose challenges on clinic staff and patients alike [42].

2.4 Application

2.4.1 Colorectal cancer screening

Colorectal cancer initiates in the colon, the extended tube responsible for transporting digested food to the rectum and eventually out of the body. This cancer arises from specific polyps or growths in the inner lining of the colon. Healthcare providers employ screening tests to identify precancerous polyps before they transform into cancerous tumors. Screening colonoscopy offers potential benefits to patients in two ways. Primarily, it can identify and facilitate the removal of precancerous polyps. Additionally, colonoscopy has the capability to detect cancers at an early stage, increasing the likelihood of successful treatment compared to those found in more advanced stages. Given its ability to detect and remove polyps before they progress to cancer, colonoscopy appears to be an ideal screening tool [43, 44].

2.4.2 Gastrointestinal perforation

A gastrointestinal perforation is a severe condition necessitating immediate medical attention. Specific medical conditions and injuries can increase the likelihood of experiencing gastrointestinal perforation. However, with swift medical intervention, many individuals achieve a complete recovery. A colonoscopy is essential for providing interior images of the large intestine or colon [45].

2.4.3 Chronic colitis such as Crohn's disease or ulcerative colitis

The digestive system becomes inflamed and irritated when an individual has Crohn's disease. Abdominal discomfort, diarrhea, loss of weight, and rectal bleeding are possible symptoms. While this condition is lifelong and currently incurable, available treatments are generally effective in symptom management, enabling an active lifestyle. Colonoscopy is a commonly used diagnostic tool, involving the use of a colonoscope, a thin tube with a light and camera attachment to examine the interior of the colon. Additionally, the doctor might conduct a biopsy, extracting a tissue sample from the colon to check for signs of inflammation. Ulcerative colitis (UC) is a chronic condition characterized by inflammation and ulcers within the colon (large intestine). As a prevalent form of IBD, UC frequently leads to symptoms such as bloody diarrhea and abdominal cramping. In the diagnostic process, a colonoscopy is performed using a slender, flexible tube equipped with a tiny camera. The endoscope is inserted through the rectum by a healthcare provider to examine the interior of the colon and collect tissue samples for biopsy testing [46].

2.4.4 Colonic ischemia

Colonic ischemia is a condition that arises when there is partial or complete blockage of blood flow to the colon. Typically, the blockage occurs in one or more arteries that supply blood to the large intestine. Colonic ischemia can manifest either acutely, with a sudden onset, or chronically, developing gradually over time. This disorder is more prevalent in older individuals, particularly those with cardiovascular diseases or blood clotting disorders. Colonoscopy is a common diagnostic method for detecting ischemia. If there is suspicion of an issue in the colon, large intestine, or the lower part of the small intestine, a colonoscope is inserted through the rectum. Colonoscopy is particularly recommended for individuals who cannot undergo a contrast injection, especially those with allergies or kidney problems [47].

2.4.5 Ischemic colitis

Ischemic colitis is a form of colitis, involving inflammation in the colon, but it differs from other types as it originates in the circulatory system. The colon experiences reduced blood flow, leading to oxygen deprivation and triggering an inflammatory response. Without the restoration of blood flow, it may result in tissue death. In cases of tissue death or rupture in the colon wall, removal of the affected part may be necessary through colonoscopy. Bowel resection, which might involve a temporary or permanent colostomy, could also be considered [48].

3. Complications related to colonoscopy

There are many complications related to colonoscopy. **Figure 2** displays the various complications related to colonoscopy.

3.1 Serious gastrointestinal colonoscopy complications

Several studies have examined the serious consequences of colonoscopies; the majority of these studies have concentrated on the risks associated with gastrointestinal bleeding or colonic perforation. Diverticulitis and postpolypectomy syndrome are two more severe side effects. At least 4 weeks after the colonoscopy, major consequences including gastrointestinal bleeding have been known to occur at delayed intervals. For this reason, it is important to monitor the rate of complications. Extensive research has focused primarily on investigating the possibility of colonic perforation. Despite being a potentially severe complication, its occurrence is infrequent, as indicated by findings from extensive studies, with reported rates generally below 0.3% and often less than 0.1%. On the other hand, the most prevalent serious complication is lower gastrointestinal bleeding, with reported risks ranging from 0.1 to 0.6% [49]. The degree of risk reduction in complications when employing colonoscopy for screening or surveillance purposes compared to diagnostic purposes remains uncertain. A comprehensive study carried out by the

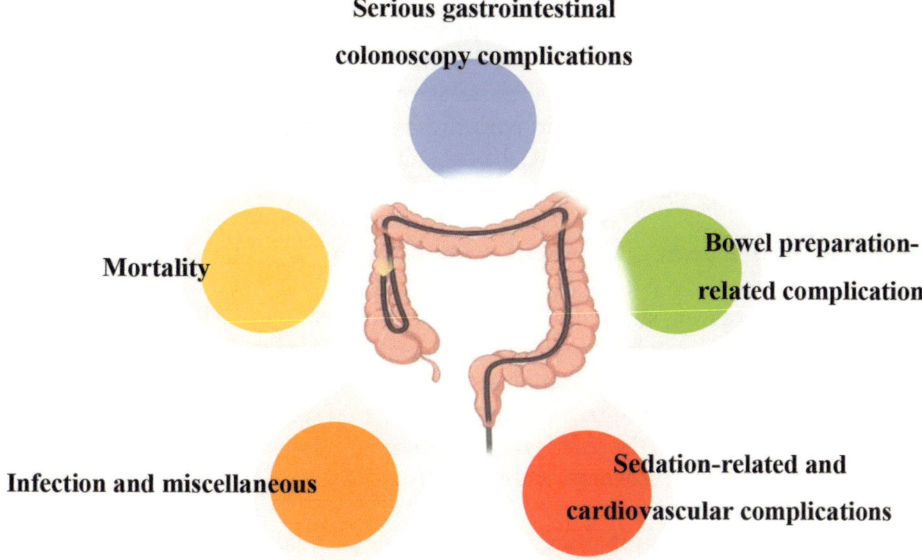

Figure 2.
Complications related to colonoscopy.

U.S. Preventive Services Task Force concluded that among mostly asymptomatic patients, the estimated incidence of significant consequences after screening colonoscopies was 2.8 per 1000 assessments [50].

3.2 Bowel preparation-related complication

Bowel preparation regimens fall into two broad categories: those based on electrolyte solutions with polyethylene glycol (PEG) and those without PEG, including sodium phosphate solutions. Although the sodium phosphate formulations with lesser volumes are usually well tolerated, there have been concerns expressed over the possibility of kidney damage with these regimens. Research on colonoscopies in healthy adults has indicated the occurrence of notable hypocalcemia or hyperphosphatemia with these preparations [51]. The possibility of acute phosphate nephropathy from calcium-phosphate crystal precipitation in the kidney is the most worrisome. Individuals who are dehydrated or old may be more susceptible to acute phosphate nephropathy. Additionally, using some antihypertensive drugs, such as diuretics, ACE inhibitors, or angiotensin receptor blockers (ARBs), may raise the risk if a person has hypertension. Although the exact risk is unclear, acute phosphate nephropathy is thought to affect fewer than 0.1% of people [52]. In a backward-looking investigation, Hurst and co-researchers identified acute kidney injury, characterized by a rise in serum creatinine exceeding 0.5 mg/dL, in 1.2% of patients within a year following colonoscopy. Compared to those who utilized PEG-based solutions, those who had undergone a sodium phosphate preparation had a greater incidence of acute renal damage [53]. It is not recommended to use sodium phosphate preparations in senior patients, people with pre-existing renal illness, or people who already have fluid or electrolyte imbalances, such as congestive heart failure patients. PEG-based treatments are thought to be safe for those with chronic renal disease, congestive cardiac failure, and electrolyte abnormalities because they do not significantly affect fluid balance. Nevertheless, due to the substantial volume of the required preparation, patients often find it challenging to tolerate [54]. Nausea and vomiting, along with a sense of abdominal fullness, are frequently experienced during the intake of large-volume preparations. Conditions such as vomiting-induced Mallory-Weiss tears, esophageal disruption, pulmonary aspiration, hypothermia, and cardiac arrhythmias are uncommon side effects associated with these preparations [55]. Imbalances in electrolytes are less frequent with PEG-based solutions in comparison to sodium phosphate preparations, as has been recorded.

3.3 Sedation-related and cardiovascular complications

Although they are rare, serious side effects from mild sedation during a colonoscopy might include hypoxia, respiratory depression, cardiac arrhythmia, hypertension, and vasovagal responses. In a meta-analysis of randomized studies for mild sedation, McQuaid and Laine discovered that patients getting midazolam alone had an 18% risk of hypoxemia, compared to those receiving midazolam plus a narcotic, who had an 11% risk [56]. Examining information derived from 174,255 colonoscopies within the Clinical Outcomes Research Initiative (CORI) database, Sharma and team identified a general incidence of cardiopulmonary complications post-colonoscopy at a rate of 1100 per 100,000 procedures [57]. The prevalent cardiopulmonary complications included transient hypoxia, bradycardia, hypotension, and vasovagal reactions. The possibility of having too many cardiovascular events within 30 days following a colonoscopy has raised more worries. When Warren and coworkers examined Medicare seniors' risk of cardiovascular events after a colonoscopy, they discovered a slightly higher risk of events needing an ER visit or hospital stay than in a sample with similar age, gender, and comorbidities [51]. Arrhythmia emerged as the prevailing adverse cardiovascular occurrence. The heightened likelihood of cardiovascular events was particularly notable in individuals who underwent a polypectomy in contrast to matched counterparts who either did not undergo colonoscopy or underwent either screening or diagnostic colonoscopy. Conditions such as diabetes, stroke, atrial fibrillation, or congestive cardiac failure have been associated with a higher likelihood of cardiovascular events as compared to people lacking these underlying medical disorders. Nevertheless, there was no statistically significant difference in the risk of cardiovascular events between the groups that were matched and the individuals who were not undergoing a colonoscopy. Another trial using screening and surveillance colonoscopies, including individuals who were generally younger, did not find a greater chance of cardiovascular episodes.

3.4 Infection

Following colonoscopy, whether with or without polypectomy, a temporary presence of bacteria in the bloodstream happens in roughly 4% of procedures, with variability in the range of occurrence from 0–25% [58]. Inflammation stemming from conditions such as toxic megacolon, fulminant colitis, ulcerative colitis, Crohn's flares, diverticulitis, and others may arise. Although isolated instances of infection subsequent to colonoscopy have been documented, there was no established direct causative connection with the endoscopic procedure. Moreover, there was no confirmed advantage associated with antibiotic prophylaxis. As a result, both the American Heart Association and ASGE currently discourage patients having colonoscopies from using antibiotic prophylaxis [59].

3.5 Mortality

Fatal incidents associated with colonoscopy, with or without polypectomy, have been infrequently documented. Out of 371,099 colonoscopies, a 2010 study found 128 recorded fatalities related to the procedure. The study encompassed both prospective research and retrospective examination of large clinical or administrative datasets. An overall unweighted mortality rate of 0.03% was the result of this [49]. While some investigation recorded death from all causes, and others restricted their analysis to mortality specifically related to colonoscopy, all studies documented mortality within 30 days following the procedure.

3.6 Miscellaneous complication

Severe appendicitis, incarcerated hernias, subcutaneous emphysema without perforation, intramural hematoma, and ischemic colitis are uncommon and infrequent problems related to colonoscopies. Instances of colonic explosions have been documented in patients undergoing electrocautery, especially those with inadequate bowel preparation, notably with mannitol preparations, although the latter are not presently in use [60]. While it is common to experience temporary bacteremia during a colonoscopy, antibiotic prophylaxis is not usually advised due to the rarity of bacteremia consequences such as infective endocarditis. Glutaraldehyde endoscopic disinfection may cause a chemical colitis if the endoscope is not completely cleansed before the start of the procedure.

4. Risk factors

A major risk factor for major gastrointestinal problems following a colonoscopy has repeatedly been demonstrated to be growing older. In contrast to patients aged 65–69 years, Gatto and colleagues observed that subjects aged 75–79 years old had a roughly fourfold higher risk of perforation [61]. The likelihood of colonic perforation, specifically, may be higher in females. This correlation may be explained by the finding that women often have more difficult colonoscopies than men do, possibly as a result of differences in pelvic anatomy and a greater frequency of previous pelvic procedures in women. In the Medicare population, the co-occurrence of concurrent conditions such as stroke, diabetes, atrial fibrillation, and congestive cardiac failure has been associated with an increased risk of major adverse outcomes; however, not all studies have shown this correlation [62]. The likelihood of complications significantly rises in procedures involving a polypectomy, especially when electrocautery is employed. Levin and co-researchers discovered a ninefold increase in the overall risk of serious complications in colonoscopies involving biopsy or polypectomy, although the risk specifically related to perforation did not show a significant increase. Furthermore, the risk of complications, predominantly gastrointestinal bleeding, escalates even more when multiple polypectomies with electrocautery are performed [63]. Complications may also arise from a biopsy alone. Previous research has indicated that hot biopsy, especially when performed in the proximal colon, may increase the risk of bleeding when polyps are removed [64]. While certain researchers propose that the experience and proficiency of endoscopists might impact the rates of complications, there is limited data to either support or contradict this notion. In Canada, the specific expertise of the endoscopist did not impact the chances of complications. However, endoscopists who performed fewer colonoscopies had a higher risk of complications compared to those who performed a higher number of procedures. It is worth noting that when considering only colonoscopies conducted by gastroenterologists, the volume of colonoscopies was not linked to the risk of complications [62]. Complications from colonoscopies may also be more likely in those taking clopidogrel or warfarin [65]. For example, Hui and colleagues found that the risk of postpolypectomy bleeding was higher when warfarin was used, even after considering factors such as the age of the patient, polyp position and dimensions, polypectomy technique, and underlying renal impairment. On the other hand, there is no evidence that taking aspirin or nonsteroidal anti-inflammatory drugs increases the likelihood of postpolypectomy bleeding [66]. According to the guidelines from the American Society of Gastrointestinal Endoscopy, individuals having endoscopic treatments may not necessarily need to stop taking aspirin or nonsteroidal anti-inflammatory medicines. The underlying indications for clopidogrel's use as well as the potential dangers associated with the scheduled surgery must be taken into consideration while making decisions regarding stopping the medication.

5. Management of complications related to colonoscopy

5.1 Patient management

Any patient who encounters a problem needs to be attended to right away by skilled medical professionals, who frequently comprise a multidisciplinary team including surgeons, interventional radiologists, and endoscopists. Typically, surgical consultation is recommended as well. Patients should be admitted right away to an institution that is prepared to handle problems that do not respond to urgent colonoscopic care. These complications may need medical, surgical, radiologic, or other therapies [67]. While many complications in medical procedures are inevitable, some do result from errors in healthcare. In recent times, there has been a growing focus on providing patients with information about medical mistakes. These mistakes are described by the Institute of Medicine as either the failure to carry out a planned action as intended or the use of an incorrect plan to achieve a goal. Studies indicate a disparity between patients' expectations regarding the disclosure and apology for medical errors and the actual proficiency of physicians in effectively communicating such errors. Consequently, numerous institutions are adopting policies mandating the disclosure of medical errors. Since 2001, the Joint Commission has enforced a requirement for hospitals and healthcare organizations to disclose "unanticipated outcomes" as an integral part of their accreditation standards [68]. Quality improvement initiatives should make targeted attempts to recognize adverse events occurring within 30 days following colonoscopy. Thorough evaluations of all potential issues should be carried out and deliberated among healthcare professionals in a structured environment focused on improving quality, such as a death and morbidity conference. This platform should facilitate open discussions among physicians about the procedure, enabling the identification of any aspects of care that could be enhanced. Additionally, these conferences serve to pinpoint systemic issues that, when addressed, can contribute to an improvement in the overall quality of care [69]. Both the patient group and the kind of operation being done have an impact on the likelihood of problems.

5.2 The function of specialized organizations is to minimize complications

Specific risk factors for problems are hard to identify for a particular endoscopist or small team of endoscopists because of the uncommon nature of problems and the diverse patient demographics. As a result, although each endoscopist is accountable for their own patient care, the entire group of endoscopists is collectively responsible for setting practice guidelines that maximize the advantages of colonoscopy and reduce the risk of damage to any patients. One example is the controversial and evolving topic of managing antithrombotic medications (such as warfarin, clopidogrel, and aspirin) during the time of a colonoscopy. Professional associations for gastroenterology have updated their guidelines in response to new data on the risks of blood clot-related events versus the hazards of bleeding problems from discontinuing antithrombotic medical care [70]. Specialized societies in gastroenterology have proactively engaged in educating their members about recognized issues and the corresponding corrective measures. They have also been involved in formulating and revising guidelines for the reprocessing of endoscopes and associated equipment. It is essential for these specialty societies to persist in promoting rigorous standards for endoscopist training and supporting ongoing research aimed at preventing complications arising from colonoscopies [71]. Patents related to the colonoscopy are given in **Table 1**.

6. Conclusion and future scope

Artificial intelligence (AI) is becoming more widespread, and its application to healthcare is developing quickly. AI is being investigated widely in the field of cancer

Sr. no	Title	Patent number
1	Methods, systems, and media for simultaneously monitoring colonoscopic video quality and detecting polyps in colonoscopy	US10861151B2
2	Kit comprising an osmotic laxative and a stimulant laxative for preparing the colon for virtual colonoscopy	EP1976520B1
3	Hydro-colonoscopy combination system	US20130245380A1
4	Crohn's disease assistant diagnosis system and method under a kind of colonoscopy based on deep learning	CN109615633A
5	Ulcerative colitis assistant diagnosis system and method under colonoscopy based on deep learning	CN109447987A
6	Edible semi-solid composition for use in patients undergoing endoscopy including colonoscopy	US20190298757A1
7	Method and apparatus for real-time detection of polyps in optical colonoscopy	EP3479348B1

Table 1.
Patent search analytical report.

screening to help interpret imaging tests such as mammography for breast cancer and colonoscopy for colorectal cancer. The overall number of adenomas found did increase as a result of the screening procedure's implementation of computer-aided diagnosis (CAD). However, the main cause of the increase was the discovery of much smaller growths, which are less likely to become cancer. With the development of imaging technologies, there is a possibility that the number of small adenomas detected would rise. This could potentially harm the cost efficiency of colonoscopy by raising the costs related to polypectomy and pathology, without necessarily enhancing its effectiveness. A possible strategy in addressing this advancement is to overlook small adenomatous lesions, yet the inherent capability of colonoscopy lies in its ability to identify and remove precancerous lesions simultaneously. Another option would involve identifying and eliminating small adenomas, coupled with broadening the category of adenomas deemed low risk. This could lead to longer intervals for postpolypectomy monitoring, possibly up to 10 years or more, particularly if the examination includes thorough removal of even the tiniest and flattest lesions. The expense associated with evaluating pathology for very small polyps is considerable, and the primary purpose of pathologically assessing polyps measuring 5 mm or less is to determine postpolypectomy surveillance intervals. If effective methods for examining polyp tissue in actual time were developed, it would be possible to remove or cut out small polyps and discard them. Afterward, follow-up monitoring after polyp removal could depend on immediate endoscopic assessment of tissue characteristics. The significant financial benefits from this progress would enhance the overall cost efficiency of colonoscopy and polypectomy in comparison to other imaging methods [72]. The extent to which anesthesia specialists participate in colonoscopy sedation will significantly influence the overall cost-effectiveness of colonoscopy in comparison to alternative diagnostic imaging strategies. In the coming years, colonoscopy is expected to be the favored diagnostic method for people with positive screening results and those displaying symptoms strongly suggestive of colorectal cancer. These symptoms may include hemochromatemia, deficiencies in iron, and melena, particularly when an upper endoscopy reveals no abnormalities [73]. Hence, the exploration of any potential progress in addressing the factors contributing to interval cancers is deemed worthwhile. As mentioned previously, the widespread adoption of strategies to enhance the effectiveness and safety of colonoscopies, coupled with advancements in colonoscope technology, is expected to strengthen the role of colonoscopy as a leading primary screening method compared to emerging imaging technologies. Beyond readily attainable improvements, it is important to note that colonoscopy is evolving, and innovations in imaging and potential insertion platforms could further enhance its efficacy and cost-effectiveness [74].

Author details

Riya Patel*, Shivani Patel, Ilyas Momin and Shreeraj Shah
LJ Institute of Pharmacy, LJ University, LJ Campus, Ahmedabad, India

*Address all correspondence to: riaapatel13@gmail.com

References

[1] Stauffer CM, Pfeifer C. Colonoscopy. Treasure Island (FL): StatPearls Publishing; 2023. pp. 1-12

[2] Anderson JC, Messina CR, Cohn W, Gottfried E, Ingber S, Bernstein G, et al. Factors predictive of difficult colonoscopy. Gastrointestinal Endoscopy. 2001;**54**:558-562. DOI: 10.1067/MGE.2001.118950

[3] Siegel RL, Miller KD, Jemal A. Cancer statistics. CA: A Cancer Journal for Clinicians. 2018;**68**:7-30. DOI: 10.3322/caac.21442

[4] Hayman CV, Vyas D. Screening colonoscopy: The present and the future. World Journal of Gastroenterology. 2021;**27**:233-239. DOI: 10.3748/WJG.V27.I3.233

[5] Fu L, Dai M, Liu J, Shi H, Pan J, Lan Y, et al. Study on the influence of assistant experience on the quality of colonoscopy: A pilot single-center study. Medicine. 2019;**98**:e17747. DOI: 10.1097/MD.0000000000017747

[6] Roy PS, Saikia BJ. Cancer and cure: A critical analysis. Indian Journal of Cancer. 2016;**53**:441-442. DOI: 10.4103/0019-509X.200658

[7] Winawer SJ. The history of colorectal cancer screening: A personal perspective. Digestive Diseases and Sciences. 2015;**60**:596-608. DOI: 10.1007/s10620-014-3466-y

[8] Amlani B, Radaelli F, Bhandari P. A survey on colonoscopy shows poor understanding of its protective value and widespread misconceptions across Europe. PLoS One. 2020;**15**:1-13. DOI: 10.1371/journal.pone.0233490

[9] Rastogi A, Wani S. Colonoscopy. Gastrointestinal Endoscopy. 2017;**85**:59-66. DOI: 10.1016/j.gie.2016.09.013

[10] Rees CJ, Thomas Gibson S, Rutter MD, Baragwanath P, Pullan R, Feeney M, et al. UK key performance indicators and quality assurance standards for colonoscopy. Gut. 2016;**65**:1923-1929. DOI: 10.1136/gutjnl-2016-312044

[11] Ahlquist DA, Hara AK, Johnson CD. Computed tomographic colography and virtual colonoscopy. Gastrointestinal Endoscopy Clinics of North America. 1997;**7**:439-452. DOI: 10.1016/s1052-5157(18)30298-8

[12] P.A.N. Gastroenterology, National Naval Medical Center; the Department of Radiology, F. Edward Hébert School of Medicine. Uniformed Services University of the Health Sciences. The New England Journal of Medicine. 2003;**23**:2191-2200

[13] Agha M, Mansy H, Ellatif HA. Virtual colonoscopy: Technical guide to avoid traps and pitfalls. Egyptian Journal of Radiology and Nuclear Medicine. 2016;**47**:17-31. DOI: 10.1016/j.ejrnm.2015.12.001

[14] Stoffel EM, Turgeon DK, Stockwell DH, Normolle DP, Tuck MK, Marcon NE, et al. Chromoendoscopy detects more adenomas than colonoscopy using intensive inspection without dye spraying. Cancer Prevention Research. 2008;**1**:507-513. DOI: 10.1158/1940-6207.CAPR-08-0096

[15] Galloro G, Ruggiero S, Russo T, Saunders B. Recent advances to improve the endoscopic detection and differentiation of early colorectal neoplasia. Colorectal Disease. 2015;**17**:25-30. DOI: 10.1111/codi.12818

[16] Ahmed R, Santhirakumar K, Butt H, Yetisen AK. Colonoscopy technologies for diagnostics and drug delivery. Medical Devices & Sensors. 2019;**2**:1-16. DOI: 10.1002/mds3.10041

[17] Kahi CJ. Chromocolonoscopy for colorectal cancer screening: Dive into the big blue. Journal of Interventional Gastroenterology. 2012;**2**:112-113. DOI: 10.4161/jig.23729

[18] Wu L, Li P, Wu J, Cao Y, Gao F. The diagnostic accuracy of chromoendoscopy for dysplasia in ulcerative colitis: Meta-analysis of six randomized controlled trials. Colorectal Disease. 2012;**14**:416-420. DOI: 10.1111/j.1463-1318.2010.02505.x

[19] Vişovan II, Tanţău M, Pascu O, Ciobanu L, Tanţău A. The role of narrow band imaging in colorectal polyp detection. Bosnian Journal of Basic Medical Sciences. 2017;**17**:152-158. DOI: 10.17305/bjbms.2017.1686

[20] Gromski MA, Kahi CJ. Advanced colonoscopy techniques and technologies. Techniques in Gastrointestinal Endoscopy. 2015;**17**:192-198. DOI: 10.1016/j.tgie.2016.01.003

[21] Yamashina T, Takeuchi Y, Uedo N, Aoi K, Matsuura N, Nagai K, et al. Diagnostic features of sessile serrated adenoma/polyps on magnifying narrow band imaging: A prospective study of diagnostic accuracy. Journal of Gastroenterology and Hepatology (Australia). 2015;**30**:117-123. DOI: 10.1111/jgh.12688

[22] Patel G, Patel R. Chapter 11 - Thermoresponsive hydrogel: A carrier for tissue engineering and regenerative medicine. In: Oliveira JM, Silva-Correia J, Reis RL, editors. Hydrogels for Tissue Engineering and Regenerative Medicine. Portugal, Europe: Academic Press; 2024. pp. 213-232. DOI: 10.1016/B978-0-12-823948-3.00009-9

[23] Subramanian V, Ragunath K. Advanced endoscopic imaging: A review of commercially available technologies. Clinical Gastroenterology and Hepatology. 2014;**12**:368-376.e1. DOI: 10.1016/j.cgh.2013.06.015

[24] Patel G, Patel P, Sonara Z, Patel R. Fabrication and optimization of 3d printed insert coated with rate controlling membrane in the treatment of recurrent vaginal candidiasis via vaginal route. Social Science Research Network. United States: NYC; 2023. DOI: 10.2139/SSRN.4514316

[25] Yoshida N, Naito Y, Inada Y, Kugai M, Inoue K, Uchiyama K, et al. The detection of surface patterns by flexible spectral imaging color enhancement without magnification for diagnosis of colorectal polyps. International Journal of Colorectal Disease. 2012;**27**:605-611. DOI: 10.1007/s00384-011-1380-8

[26] Lami G, Galli A, Biagini MR, Tarocchi M, Milani S, Polvani S. Gastric and duodenal polyps in familial adenomatous polyposis patients: Conventional endoscopy vs virtual chromoendoscopy (fujinon intelligent color enhancement) in dysplasia evaluation. World Journal of Clinical Oncology. 2017;**8**:168-177. DOI: 10.5306/wjco.v8.i2.168

[27] Osawa H, Yamamoto H. Present and future status of flexible spectral imaging color enhancement and blue laser imaging technology. Digestive Endoscopy. 2014;**26**(Suppl. 1):105-115. DOI: 10.1111/den.12205

[28] Shah S, Patel R, Patel G. Nanocomposite hydrogels: An optimistic insight towards the treatments of ocular disorders. Recent Patents on Nanotechnology. 2023;**17**:89-150

[29] Cho JH. Advanced imaging technology other than narrow band imaging. Clinical Endoscopy. 2015;**48**:503-510. DOI: 10.5946/ce.2015.48.6.503

[30] Patel S, Jha LL. Application of Plackett-Burman and box-Behnken designs for screening and optimization of Rotigotine Hcl and rasagiline mesylate transfersomes: A statistical approach. International Journal of Applied Pharmaceutics. 2023;**15**:238-245. DOI: 10.22159/ijap.2023v15i4.47674

[31] Patel SM, Jha LL. Simultaneous UV method development for determination of rotigotine hydrochloride and rasagiline mesylate. Indian Drugs. 2023;**60**:73-79. DOI: 10.53879/id.60.05.13373

[32] Bowman EA, Pfau PR, Mitra A, Reichelderfer M, Gopal DV, Hall BS, et al. High definition colonoscopy combined with i-SCAN imaging technology is superior in the detection of adenomas and advanced lesions compared to high definition colonoscopy alone. Diagnostic and Therapeutic Endoscopy. 2015;**2015**:167406. DOI: 10.1155/2015/167406

[33] Patel RJ, Pandey P, Patel AA, Prajapati BG, Alexander A, Pandya V, et al. Ordered mesoporous silica nanocarriers: An innovative paradigm and a promising therapeutic efficient carrier for delivery of drugs. Journal of Drug Delivery Science and Technology. 2023;**82**:104306. DOI: 10.1016/j.jddst.2023.104306

[34] Shah S, Patel AA, Prajapati BG, Alexander A, Pandya V, Trivedi N, et al. Multifaceted nanolipidic carriers: A modish stratagem accentuating nose-to-brain drug delivery. Journal of Nanoparticle Research. 2023;**25**:1-34. DOI: 10.1007/s11051-023-05804-4

[35] Hoffman A, Sar F, Goetz M, Tresch A, Mudter J, Biesterfeld S, et al. High definition colonoscopy combined with i-scan is superior in the detection of colorectal neoplasias compared with standard video colonoscopy: A prospective randomized controlled trial. Endoscopy. 2010;**42**:827-833. DOI: 10.1055/s-0030-1255713

[36] Fujiya M, Kohgo Y. Image-enhanced endoscopy for the diagnosis of colon neoplasms. Gastrointestinal Endoscopy. 2013;**77**:111-118.e5. DOI: 10.1016/j.gie.2012.07.031

[37] Takeuchi Y, Inoue T, Hanaoka N, Higashino K, Iishi H, Chatani R, et al. Autofluorescence imaging with a transparent hood for detection of colorectal neoplasms: A prospective, randomized trial. Gastrointestinal Endoscopy. 2010;**72**:1006-1013. DOI: 10.1016/j.gie.2010.06.055

[38] Patel R, Shah U, Patel G. Optimization of poly (E-caprolactone) based biodegradable in situ porous drug-eluting insert of BCS class II/IV drug for targeted application. International Journal of Polymeric Materials and Polymeric Biomaterials. 2023;**73**:1-12. DOI: 10.1080/00914037.2023.2222334

[39] Yung DE, Rondonotti E, Koulaouzidis A. Review: Capsule colonoscopy-a concise clinical overview of current status. Annals of Translational Medicine. 2016;**4**:398. DOI: 10.21037/atm.2016.10.71

[40] Spada C, Pasha SF, Gross SA, Leighton JA, Schnoll-Sussman F, Correale L, et al. Accuracy of first- and second-generation colon capsules in endoscopic detection of colorectal polyps: A systematic review and meta-analysis. Clinical Gastroenterology and Hepatology. 2016;**14**:1533-1543.e8. DOI: 10.1016/j.cgh.2016.04.038

[41] Alarcón-Fernández O, Ramos L, Adrián-de-Ganzo Z, Gimeno-García AZ,

Nicolás-Pérez D, Jiménez A, et al. Effects of colon capsule endoscopy on medical decision making in patients with incomplete colonoscopies. Clinical Gastroenterology and Hepatology. 2013;**11**:534-540.e1. DOI: 10.1016/j.cgh.2012.10.016

[42] Patel R, Shah R, Patel A, Hadiya K, Parmar J, Patel G. Off-label use of raloxifene hydrochloride in uterine fibroids: A novel insert-based formulation approach and *in-vivo* preclinical evaluation. Journal of Drug Delivery Science and Technology. 2023;**84**:104552. DOI: 10.1016/j.jddst.2023.104552

[43] Young PE, Womeldorph CM. Colonoscopy for colorectal cancer screening. Journal of Cancer. 2013;**4**:217-226. DOI: 10.7150/jca.5829

[44] Patel R, Yadav BK, Patel G. Progresses in nano-enabled platforms for the treatment of vaginal disorders. Recent Patents on Nanotechnology. 2022;**17**:208-227. DOI: 10.2174/1872210516666220628150447

[45] Anderson ML, Pasha TM, Leighton JA. Endoscopic perforation of the colon: Lessons from a 10-year study. American Journal of Gastroenterology. 2000;**95**:3418-3422. DOI: 10.1016/S0002-9270(00)02149-3

[46] García-Bosch O, Ordás I, Aceituno M, Rodríguez S, Ramírez AM, Gallego M, et al. Comparison of diagnostic accuracy and impact of magnetic resonance imaging and colonoscopy for the management of Crohn's disease. Journal of Crohn's and Colitis. 2016;**10**:663-669. DOI: 10.1093/ecco- jcc/jjw015

[47] Sadalla S, Lisotti A, Fuccio L, Fusaroli P. Colonoscopy-related colonic ischemia. World Journal of Gastroenterology. 2021;**27**:7299-7310. DOI: 10.3748/wjg.v27.i42.7299

[48] Lozano-Maya M, Ponferrada-Díaz A, González-Asanza C, Nogales-Rincón O, Senent-Sánchez C, Pérez-de-Ayala V, et al. Usefulness of colonoscopy in ischemic colitis. Revista Espanola de Enfermedades Digestivas. 2010;**102**:478-483. DOI: 10.4321/S1130- 01082010000800004

[49] Ko CW, Dominitz JA. Complications of colonoscopy: Magnitude and management. Gastrointestinal Endoscopy Clinics of North America. 2010;**20**:659-671. DOI: 10.1016/j.giec.2010.07.005

[50] Adult R, Schedule I, States U. Annals of internal medicine clinical guidelines changes in the schedule. Annals of Internal Medicine. 2008;**147**:1-5

[51] Warren JL, Klabunde CN, Mariotto AB, Meekins A, Topor M, Brown ML, et al. Adverse events after outpatient colonoscopy in the medicare population. Annals of Internal Medicine. 2009;**150**:849-857. DOI: 10.7326/0003-4819-150-12-200906160-00008

[52] Markowitz GS, Radhakrishnan J, D'Agati VD. Towards the incidence of acute phosphate nephropathy. Journal of the American Society of Nephrology. 2007;**18**:3020-3022. DOI: 10.1681/ASN.2007101073

[53] Hurst FP, Bohen EM, Osgard EM, Oliver DK, Das NP, Gao SW, et al. Association of oral sodium phosphate purgative use with acute kidney injury. Journal of the American Society of Nephrology. 2007;**18**:3192-3198. DOI: 10.1681/ASN.2007030349

[54] Hawes RH, Lowry A, Deziel D. Preamble. Gastrointestinal Endoscopy. 2006;**63**:894. DOI: 10.1016/j.gie.2006.03.919

[55] Adamcewicz M, Bearelly D, Porat G, Friedenberg FK. Mechanism

of action and toxicities of purgatives used for colonoscopy preparation. Expert Opinion on Drug Metabolism and Toxicology. 2011;7:89-101. DOI: 10.1517/17425255.2011.542411

[56] McQuaid KR, Laine L. A systematic review and meta-analysis of randomized, controlled trials of moderate sedation for routine endoscopic procedures. Gastrointestinal Endoscopy. 2008;**67**:910-923. DOI: 10.1016/j.gie.2007.12.046

[57] Sharma VK, Nguyen CC, Crowell MD, Lieberman DA, de Garmo P, Fleischer DE. A national study of cardiopulmonary unplanned events after GI endoscopy {a figure is presented}. Gastrointestinal Endoscopy. 2007;**66**:27-34. DOI: 10.1016/j.gie.2006.12.040

[58] Nelson DB. Infectious disease complications of GI endoscopy: Part II, exogenous infections. Gastrointestinal Endoscopy. 2003;**57**:695-711. DOI: 10.1067/mge.2003.202

[59] Wilson W, Taubert KA, Gewitz M, Lockhart PB, Baddour LM, Levison M, et al. Prevention of infective endocarditis: Guidelines from the American Heart Association. Circulation. 2007;**116**:1736-1754. DOI: 10.1161/CIRCULATIONAHA.106.183095

[60] Bigard MA, Gaucher P, Lassalle C. Fatal colonic explosion during colonoscopic polypectomy. Gastroenterology. 1979;**77**:1307-1310. DOI: 10.1016/0016-5085(79)90172-0

[61] Schoen RE, Levin TR, Gatto NM, Neugut AI, Frucht H. Re: Risk of perforation after colonoscopy and sigmoidoscopy: A population-based study (multiple letters) [3]. Journal of the National Cancer Institute. 2003;**95**:830-831. DOI: 10.1093/jnci/95.11.830-a

[62] Rabeneck L, Paszat LF, Hilsden RJ, Saskin R, Leddin D, Grunfeld E, et al. Bleeding and perforation after outpatient colonoscopy and their risk factors in usual clinical practice. Gastroenterology. 2008;**135**:1899-1906.e1. DOI: 10.1053/j.gastro.2008.08.058

[63] Stockman JA. Complications of colonoscopy in an integrated health care delivery system. Yearbook of Pediatrics. 2008;**2008**:167-168. DOI: 10.1016/s0084-3954(08)70370-1

[64] Dyer WS, Quigley EMM, Noel SM, Camacho KE, Manela F, Zetterman RK. Major colonic hemorrhage following electrocoagulating (hot) biopsy of diminutive colonic polyps: Relationship to colonic location and low-dose aspirin therapy. Gastrointestinal Endoscopy. 1991;**37**:361-364. DOI: 10.1016/S0016-5107(91)70733-5

[65] Hui AJ, Wong RMY, Ching JYL, Hung LCT, Chung SCS, Sung JJY. Risk of colonoscopic polypectomy bleeding with anticoagulants and antiplatelet agents: Analysis of 1657 cases. Gastrointestinal Endoscopy. 2004;**59**:44-48. DOI: 10.1016/S0016-5107(03)02307-1

[66] Shiffman ML, Farrel MT, Yee YS. Risk of bleeding after endoscopic biopsy or polypectomy in patients taking aspirin or other NSAIDs. Gastrointestinal Endoscopy. 1994;**40**:458-462. DOI: 10.1016/S0016-5107(94)70210-1

[67] Panteris V, Haringsma J, Kuipers EJ. Colonoscopy perforation rate, mechanisms and outcome: From diagnostic to therapeutic colonoscopy. Endoscopy. 2009;**41**:941-951. DOI: 10.1055/s-0029-1215179

[68] Hendee WR. To err is human: Building a safer health system. Journal of Vascular and Interventional Radiology.

2001;**12**:112-P113. DOI: 10.1016/s1051-0443(01)70072-3

[69] Hasan AG, Brown WR. A model for mortality-morbidity conferences in gastroenterology. Gastrointestinal Endoscopy. 2008;**67**:515-518. DOI: 10.1016/j.gie.2007.07.006

[70] Anderson MA, Ben-Menachem T, Gan SI, Appalaneni V, Banerjee S, Cash BD, et al. Management of antithrombotic agents for endoscopic procedures. Gastrointestinal Endoscopy. 2009;**70**:1060-1070. DOI: 10.1016/j.gie.2009.09.040

[71] Banerjee S, Shen B, Nelson DB, Lichtenstein DR, Baron TH, Anderson MA, et al. Infection control during GI endoscopy. Gastrointestinal Endoscopy. 2008;**67**:781-790. DOI: 10.1016/j.gie.2008.01.027

[72] Rex DK, Helbig CC. High yields of small and flat adenomas with high-definition colonoscopes using either white light or narrow band imaging. Gastroenterology. 2007;**133**:42-47. DOI: 10.1053/j.gastro.2007.04.029

[73] Pan J, Xin L, Ma YF, Hu LH, Li ZS. Colonoscopy reduces colorectal cancer incidence and mortality in patients with non-malignant findings: A meta-analysis. American Journal of Gastroenterology. 2016;**111**:355-365. DOI: 10.1038/ajg.2015.418

[74] Rösch T, Adler A, Pohl H, Wettschureck E, Koch M, Wiedenmann B, et al. A motor-driven single-use colonoscope controlled with a hand-held device: A feasibility study in volunteers. Gastrointestinal Endoscopy. 2008;**67**:1139-1146. DOI: 10.1016/j.gie.2007.10.065